# CAYENNE PEPPER MIRACLES

Unlocking Nature's potential for wellness, pain relief and vitality with cayenne pepper

## BY TERESA MILLER

# TABLE OF CONTENTS

# INTRODUCTION

In the realm of herbal remedies, few ingredients wield the fiery vigor and versatile healing prowess quite like cayenne pepper. Originating from the sun-soaked lands of Central and South America, this vibrant spice has transcended culinary boundaries to emerge as a powerhouse in traditional medicine and holistic healing practices worldwide.

Cayenne pepper, scientifically known as Capsicum annuum, traces its roots back thousands of years to the tropical regions of the Americas. Revered by ancient civilizations like the Aztecs and Mayans, this slender red pod encasing a fiery array of capsaicinoids, boasts a rich historical tapestry. Its migration through history led to its cultivation in various continents, eventually spreading its therapeutic warmth across diverse cultures.

What sets cayenne pepper apart is not just its tantalizing heat but also its remarkable medicinal properties. Beyond its role as a zesty spice in cuisines worldwide, it has long been revered for its multifaceted healing abilities. Harnessing the power of capsaicin, the compound responsible for its spiciness, cayenne pepper serves as a cornerstone in herbal medicine, addressing an extensive array of health concerns.

Within the realm of herbal remedies, cayenne pepper emerges as a transformative agent, boasting an impressive array of therapeutic applications. From digestive health to cardiovascular support, pain relief to topical remedies, this vibrant spice stands as a testament to nature's bountiful gifts to holistic wellness enthusiasts.

In herbal medicine, cayenne pepper transcends its culinary identity, offering solutions to an extensive spectrum of health issues. Its rich composition of vitamins, antioxidants, and capsaicin facilitates improved circulation, aids in digestion, and serves as a potent anti-inflammatory agent, among a myriad of other benefits.

Embark on a journey with us as we unravel the hidden gems of cayenne pepper's healing potential. Delve into its historical significance, explore its chemical composition, and discover a treasure trove of herbal remedies harnessing the fiery essence of this potent spice.

# CHAPTER ONE

## WHAT IS CAYENNE PEPPER?

Cayenne pepper is a type of chili pepper belonging to the Capsicum annuum species. It is a pungent spice derived from dried and ground red chili peppers. Known for its vibrant red color and intense heat, cayenne pepper is widely used in culinary dishes to add spiciness and flavor.

The spice derives its fiery heat primarily from a compound called capsaicin, which is found in the seeds and membranes of the pepper. The level of heat in cayenne pepper is measured on the Scoville Heat Scale, with higher Scoville units indicating greater spiciness.

Beyond its culinary uses, cayenne pepper has been highly valued for its medicinal properties for centuries. It contains various vitamins, minerals, and antioxidants, and its active component, capsaicin, has been studied for its potential health benefits. Cayenne pepper is often used in traditional herbal medicine and natural remedies for its purported abilities to aid digestion, boost metabolism, alleviate pain, and promote cardiovascular health.

Cayenne pepper is available in various forms, including whole dried peppers, powdered spice, flakes, and capsules. It is used in a wide range of cuisines globally and is also incorporated into herbal remedies, topical creams, and ointments for its potential health-promoting effects.

## THE ORIGINS OF CAYENNE PEPPER

Cayenne pepper's origins can be traced back to Central and South America. The plant belongs to the Capsicum annuum species and is believed to have originated in the region that is now known as French Guiana, in the northern part of South America.

The plant was cultivated by various indigenous cultures in the Americas for thousands of years before being introduced to other parts of the world through trade and exploration. Ancient civilizations such as the Aztecs and Mayans were known to have used chili peppers, including cayenne, both as a food spice and for medicinal purposes.

European explorers, including Christopher Columbus, encountered chili peppers during their voyages to the

Americas. These explorers were responsible for introducing chili peppers, including cayenne, to Europe and other parts of the world.

The name "cayenne" itself is derived from the city of Cayenne in French Guiana, where it was thought to have been first traded by French explorers. However, the pepper's cultivation and use spread throughout the world due to its adaptability to different climates and its popularity as a spice and herbal remedy.

Today, cayenne pepper is cultivated in various countries across the globe, including India, Mexico, the United States, and parts of Africa and Asia. Its widespread use in culinary dishes and herbal remedies has made it a staple ingredient in many cultures, contributing not only to its popularity but also to its historical and cultural significance.

Cayenne pepper possesses a variety of properties that contribute to its culinary and medicinal uses. These properties stem from its chemical composition, particularly the presence of capsaicinoids, which include capsaicin—the primary compound responsible for the pepper's heat and various health benefits. Here are some notable properties of cayenne pepper:

• Capsaicin Content: Capsaicin is the main bioactive compound in cayenne pepper. It gives the pepper its spiciness and is known for its potential health benefits, including pain relief, anti-inflammatory properties, and potential metabolism-boosting effects.

• Rich in Nutrients: Cayenne pepper is a good source of vitamins and minerals, including vitamin A, vitamin E, vitamin C, potassium, and antioxidants like carotenoids and flavonoids.

• Anti-Inflammatory: Capsaicin in cayenne pepper has shown anti-inflammatory properties, which may help alleviate inflammation-related conditions and discomfort.

• Pain Relief: Topical applications of capsaicin derived from cayenne pepper have been used traditionally to alleviate pain. It may reduce the sensitivity of pain receptors and is commonly found in over-the-counter creams for joint or muscle pain.

• Digestive Aid: Cayenne pepper is believed to stimulate saliva production and gastric juices, aiding digestion. It may also help alleviate gas and bloating.

• Metabolism Boost: Some studies suggest that capsaicin may temporarily increase metabolism and promote fat oxidation, potentially aiding in weight management.

• Cardiovascular Support: Capsaicin may have beneficial effects on heart health by promoting circulation, reducing cholesterol levels, and potentially improving blood pressure.

• Antibacterial and Antifungal Properties: Research has shown that capsaicin possesses antibacterial and antifungal properties that may help combat certain infections.

• Appetite Suppression: Capsaicin may have an impact on appetite, potentially reducing hunger and calorie intake.

• Pungency and Flavor: Beyond its health properties, cayenne pepper is used widely in cooking due to its pungent flavor, adding heat and depth to various dishes, sauces, and marinades.

It's important to note that while cayenne pepper and its active compound capsaicin offer potential health benefits, excessive consumption or application can cause irritation or adverse reactions in some individuals. Consulting with a healthcare professional before using cayenne pepper for medicinal purposes is advisable, especially for those with certain medical conditions or sensitivities.

## HEALTH BENEFITS OF CAYENNE PEPPER

Cayenne pepper is renowned for its numerous potential health benefits, owing largely to its active component, capsaicin, along with other beneficial compounds. While more research is ongoing, here are some of the reported health benefits associated with cayenne pepper:

• Pain Relief: Capsaicin has analgesic properties that can help alleviate pain. Topical creams containing capsaicin are used to relieve muscle and joint pain, including arthritis pain, by temporarily desensitizing pain receptors.

• Anti-inflammatory Effects: Capsaicin exhibits anti-inflammatory properties that may help reduce inflammation and swelling, potentially aiding in conditions like osteoarthritis and other inflammatory diseases.

• Improved Digestive Health: Cayenne pepper stimulates saliva production and digestive enzymes, aiding digestion. It may also help alleviate gas, bloating, and indigestion.

• Metabolism and Weight Management: Capsaicin may temporarily increase metabolism and promote fat oxidation, potentially assisting in weight loss by boosting calorie burning and reducing appetite.

• Heart Health: Cayenne pepper may promote heart health by improving circulation, reducing cholesterol levels, and potentially lowering blood pressure due to its vasodilatory effects.

• Antioxidant Properties: It contains antioxidants like carotenoids and flavonoids, which can help neutralize free radicals, reducing oxidative stress and supporting overall health.

• Improved Blood Circulation: Capsaicin may aid in improving blood flow by promoting the release of nitric oxide and widening blood vessels.

• Potential Anti-Cancer Effects: Some studies suggest that capsaicin may have anticancer properties by inhibiting the growth of certain cancer cells. However, further research is needed in this area.

• Relief from Nasal Congestion: Cayenne pepper may help clear nasal passages and provide relief from congestion due to its ability to stimulate secretions and promote mucus clearance.

• Antibacterial and Antifungal Properties: Capsaicin has shown antibacterial and antifungal properties that may help combat certain infections.

It's important to note that while cayenne pepper offers potential health benefits, individual reactions can vary, and excessive consumption or use may lead to irritation or adverse effects, particularly in sensitive individuals. Consulting with a healthcare professional before incorporating cayenne pepper into your diet or using it for medicinal purposes is advisable, especially if you have any underlying health conditions or concerns.

## SCIENTIFIC EVIDENCE FOR THE BENEFITS LISTED ABOVE

Below are the health benefits associated with cayenne pepper, along with scientific evidence supporting each benefit:

### Pain Relief:

Scientific Evidence: Several studies support capsaicin's role in pain relief. Research published in the "Journal of Clinical Pharmacy and Therapeutics" in 2013 showed that capsaicin patches were effective in reducing pain associated with conditions like neuropathy.

### Digestive Health:

Scientific Evidence: Studies have suggested that capsaicin may enhance gastric mucosal blood flow and stimulate saliva production and gastric secretions, potentially aiding digestion.

However, research specifically on cayenne pepper for digestive health is limited.

## Metabolism and Weight Management:

Scientific Evidence: Research indicates that capsaicin can increase energy expenditure and fat oxidation, potentially aiding weight management by temporarily boosting metabolism. A meta-analysis published in "Appetite" in 2012 suggested that capsaicinoids may help with weight maintenance.

## Cardiovascular Support:

Scientific Evidence: Capsaicin's vasodilatory effects have been studied for their potential cardiovascular benefits. A study published in "The American Journal of Clinical Nutrition" in 2009 indicated that capsaicin may improve vascular function by enhancing blood flow.

## Respiratory Health:

Scientific Evidence: Cayenne pepper's ability to clear nasal passages has not been extensively studied. However, capsaicin's role as a nasal decongestant has been investigated in some studies, though more research is needed in this specific area.

## Antioxidant Properties:

Scientific Evidence: Cayenne pepper contains antioxidants, such as carotenoids and flavonoids. A study in the "Journal of Agricultural and Food Chemistry" in 2006 found that Capsicum peppers, including cayenne, exhibited significant antioxidant activity.

## Anti-Inflammatory Effects:

Scientific Evidence: Capsaicin has shown anti-inflammatory effects in various studies. Research in the "Journal of Clinical Investigation" in 2007 indicated that capsaicin may modulate inflammatory responses by interacting with TRPV1 receptors.

## Wound Healing and Antibacterial Properties:

Scientific Evidence: Capsaicin's antibacterial properties have been explored in some studies, indicating its potential role in preventing infections. However, more research is needed specifically on cayenne pepper for wound healing.

While these studies demonstrate potential health benefits of cayenne pepper and capsaicin, further research is needed to fully understand their effects, especially concerning human clinical trials on cayenne pepper specifically. Always consult a healthcare professional before using cayenne pepper or capsaicin for medicinal purposes.

## THE USE OF CAYENNE PEPPER IN HERBAL REMEDIES

Cayenne pepper is a versatile ingredient in herbal remedies, offering a wide array of applications in traditional and alternative medicine. Its active compound, capsaicin, contributes to its therapeutic properties. Here are some common uses of cayenne pepper in herbal remedies:

• Digestive Aid: Cayenne pepper stimulates the production of saliva and gastric juices, aiding digestion. It can help relieve indigestion, gas, and bloating. A popular remedy is mixing a small amount of cayenne pepper with warm water and lemon as a digestive tonic.

• Pain Relief: Topical applications of cayenne pepper-based creams or poultices containing capsaicin can help alleviate pain associated with arthritis, muscle aches, and nerve pain. Capsaicin's ability to inhibit substance P, a neurotransmitter involved in pain perception, contributes to its analgesic effects.

• Circulation Enhancement: Cayenne pepper can enhance blood circulation by dilating blood vessels. It's used in some herbal remedies to promote cardiovascular health, prevent blood clots, and improve overall circulation.

• Cold and Flu Relief: Due to its ability to stimulate secretions and clear nasal passages, cayenne pepper is sometimes included in herbal remedies for colds and congestion. It's thought to help relieve sinus pressure and aid in breaking up mucus.

• Metabolism Booster: Capsaicin in cayenne pepper may temporarily increase metabolism and promote fat burning, contributing to weight management. Some herbalists include cayenne in formulations aimed at boosting metabolism.

• Detoxification: Cayenne pepper is occasionally used in detoxification programs to stimulate sweating and aid in toxin elimination. It's believed to support the body's natural detox processes.

• Anti-Inflammatory Properties: Cayenne's anti-inflammatory properties make it valuable in herbal remedies aimed at reducing inflammation, such as in conditions like arthritis or digestive inflammation.

• Topical Analgesic: Cayenne pepper-based creams or ointments can be applied topically to relieve localized pain, such as in sore muscles or joints.

• First Aid: In some traditional herbal medicine practices, cayenne powder is applied topically to minor cuts or wounds due to its potential antibacterial properties and ability to stop bleeding.

Remember, while cayenne pepper can offer potential benefits, its use in herbal remedies should be approached with caution. Consultation with a healthcare professional or herbalist is recommended, especially if you're considering using cayenne pepper remedies for specific health concerns or if you have any existing health conditions or sensitivities.

Cayenne pepper's chemical composition encompasses various compounds that contribute to its distinctive flavor, heat, and potential health benefits. Here are the primary components found in cayenne pepper:

• Capsaicinoids: These are the key compounds responsible for cayenne pepper's heat. Capsaicinoids include capsaicin, dihydrocapsaicin, nordihydrocapsaicin, homodihydrocapsaicin, and others. Capsaicin, in particular, is the most abundant and is associated with many of the pepper's health benefits, such as pain relief and metabolism boosting.

• Vitamins: Cayenne pepper contains vitamins, including vitamin C (ascorbic acid), vitamin E (tocopherols), vitamin K, and some B-complex vitamins like niacin (vitamin B3).

• Carotenoids: These are natural pigments responsible for the pepper's vibrant red color. Carotenoids found in cayenne pepper include beta-carotene, capsanthin, and zeaxanthin, which also act as antioxidants.

• Flavonoids: These are antioxidants found in plants that contribute to their health-promoting properties. Cayenne pepper contains flavonoids like quercetin and luteolin.

• Minerals: Cayenne pepper contains various minerals in trace amounts, including potassium, manganese, magnesium, and iron.

• Fatty Acids: Small amounts of fatty acids, such as oleic acid and linoleic acid, are present in cayenne pepper.

• Proteins and Carbohydrates: Cayenne pepper also contains proteins and carbohydrates in smaller quantities.

The chemical composition of cayenne pepper may vary slightly based on factors like the plant's variety, growing conditions, and the processing method used to prepare the spice. The presence of capsaicinoids, especially capsaicin, is a distinguishing factor in determining the pepper's heat level and many of its medicinal properties.

The combination of these compounds in cayenne pepper contributes not only to its spicy flavor but also to its potential health benefits, making it a popular ingredient in culinary dishes and herbal remedies.

Cayenne pepper is generally safe for consumption in moderate amounts, but excessive intake or sensitivity to capsaicin, its active compound, can lead to various side effects. Here are potential side effects of consuming or using cayenne pepper:

• Gastrointestinal Discomfort: Consumption of large amounts of cayenne pepper can irritate the digestive tract, leading to stomach pain, heartburn, or gastrointestinal discomfort. It may exacerbate symptoms in individuals with conditions like gastritis or ulcers.

• Irritation or Burning Sensation: Direct contact with cayenne pepper, especially in its raw form or in high concentrations, can cause skin irritation, redness, or a burning sensation. Avoid touching sensitive areas like the eyes or mucous membranes after handling cayenne pepper without washing hands thoroughly.

• Allergic Reactions: While rare, some individuals may have an allergic reaction to cayenne pepper, resulting in symptoms like hives, itching, or difficulty breathing. Seek medical attention if any allergic reactions occur.

• Exacerbation of Digestive Disorders: Individuals with gastrointestinal conditions such as irritable bowel syndrome (IBS) or inflammatory bowel disease (IBD) may experience worsened symptoms, including diarrhea or increased gut irritation, due to the spiciness of cayenne pepper.

• Increased Bleeding Risk: Cayenne pepper's ability to increase blood circulation may also lead to increased bleeding or interfere with blood clotting in some individuals. It is advisable to avoid large amounts of cayenne pepper before surgeries or if taking blood-thinning medications.

• Skin Sensitivity: Prolonged use of topical creams or ointments containing capsaicin may cause skin irritation, burning, or a sensation of warmth. It's recommended to do a patch test before widespread application and to avoid using it on broken or sensitive skin.

• Drug Interactions: Cayenne pepper supplements or high intake may interact with certain medications, affecting their effectiveness or causing adverse reactions. It's crucial to consult a healthcare professional before using cayenne pepper supplements, especially if taking medications or having underlying health conditions.

• Discomfort in Sensitive Individuals: Some individuals may experience discomfort, sweating, or flushing after consuming foods containing cayenne pepper due to its heat-producing effect.

As with any herbal remedy or supplement, moderation is key. Individuals with pre-existing medical conditions, especially digestive issues, allergies, or sensitive skin, should exercise caution when using cayenne pepper and consult a healthcare professional before incorporating it into their diet or using it for medicinal purposes.

# THE HISTORICAL USE OF CAYENNE PEPPER IN TRADITIONAL MEDICINE

Cayenne pepper has a rich history of use in traditional medicine that spans various cultures and civilizations across centuries. Here's a glimpse into the historical use of cayenne pepper in traditional medicine:

• Ancient Civilizations in the Americas: Indigenous cultures in Central and South America, including the Aztecs and Mayans, were among the first to cultivate and use cayenne pepper for both culinary and medicinal purposes. They utilized it as a remedy for digestive issues, pain relief, and to improve circulation.

• Aztec and Mayan Healing Practices: Cayenne pepper was highly esteemed in Aztec and Mayan healing practices. It was applied topically as a pain reliever and used internally to aid digestion and alleviate gastrointestinal discomfort.

• Incorporation into Ayurvedic Medicine: In Ayurvedic medicine, the traditional healing system of India, cayenne pepper was utilized for its potential to stimulate digestion, improve circulation, and support overall wellness. It was incorporated into herbal formulas for various health conditions.

• European Adoption: Cayenne pepper was introduced to Europe by explorers returning from the Americas. In traditional European herbal medicine, it was employed as a digestive aid, to promote circulation, and as a remedy for rheumatic pain.

• Colonial American Use: In North America, cayenne pepper gained popularity during the colonial period. It was valued for its ability to aid digestion, support heart health, and alleviate pain. The renowned herbalist Samuel Thomson included cayenne pepper in his herbal remedies during the 19th century.

• Traditional Chinese Medicine (TCM): Although not native to China, cayenne pepper found its way into Traditional Chinese Medicine. It was sometimes used to invigorate circulation, warm the body, and alleviate pain.

• Topical Application for Pain Relief: Across many cultures, cayenne pepper was applied topically in poultices, ointments, or plasters for its analgesic properties. It was used to relieve joint pain, muscle aches, and nerve-related pain.

Throughout history, cayenne pepper's versatility and potential medicinal properties led to its widespread adoption in various traditional healing systems. Its use ranged from treating digestive issues and pain relief to improving circulation and overall well-being. Today, its historical use continues to influence its incorporation into modern herbal remedies and alternative medicine practices.

## REMEDIES BASED ON HEALTH ISSUES

Cayenne pepper-based remedies can be categorized based on various health issues they address. Here are some common categories and the corresponding remedies:

### Pain Relief:

• Topical Pain Relief: Capsaicin-based creams or ointments for muscle pain, joint pain (such as arthritis), neuropathic pain, or headaches.

• Capsaicin Patches: Patches containing capsaicin applied to specific areas for localized pain relief.

Digestive Health:

• Digestive Tonic: Cayenne pepper mixed with warm water and lemon to aid digestion.

• Gastric Stimulant: Capsaicin's potential to stimulate gastric juices and enzymes may help with digestion.

Metabolism and Weight Management:

• Metabolism-Boosting Drinks: Cayenne pepper mixed with water, honey, or apple cider vinegar, believed to temporarily increase metabolism.

• Cayenne Pepper Supplements: Capsules or tablets containing cayenne pepper for potential weight management benefits.

Cardiovascular Support:

• Circulation-Boosting Remedies: Cayenne pepper teas or tinctures believed to improve blood circulation.

• Heart Health Formulations: Capsaicin supplements or formulations for potential cholesterol-lowering effects.

Respiratory Health:

• Congestion Relief: Capsaicin's ability to clear nasal passages used in home remedies for colds, sinus congestion, or sore throats.

Detoxification:

• Detox Drinks: Cayenne pepper mixed with other detoxifying ingredients in beverages or cleanses believed to aid detoxification.

Topical Applications:

• Pain Relieving Creams: Topical creams or salves containing capsaicin for sore muscles, joint pain, or nerve pain.

• Warming Massage Oils: Cayenne-infused oils for massages believed to provide warmth and alleviate muscle tension.

First Aid:

• Wound Healing: Cayenne powder applied topically to minor cuts or wounds for its potential antibacterial properties and ability to stop bleeding.

These categories highlight the diverse applications of cayenne pepper in addressing various health concerns. However, it's important to note that individual responses to these remedies may vary, and consulting with a healthcare professional before using cayenne pepper-based remedies, especially for specific health issues or if you have any underlying health conditions, is advisable.



## THE MEDICINAL PROPERTIES OF CAYENNE PEPPER, AS WELL AS ITS ACTIVE COMPONENTS LIKE CAPSAICIN

Cayenne pepper, enriched with various compounds, possesses a wide range of medicinal properties, largely attributed to its active component, capsaicin, and other constituents. Here's an overview of the medicinal properties of cayenne pepper, particularly highlighting capsaicin:

• Capsaicin's Analgesic Effect: Capsaicin interacts with sensory nerves, temporarily desensitizing them and reducing the perception of pain. It's used topically in creams or patches to alleviate muscle pain, joint pain (arthritis), neuropathic pain, and headaches.

• Reduction of Inflammation: Capsaicin exhibits anti-inflammatory effects by inhibiting inflammatory substances. It may help reduce inflammation in conditions like osteoarthritis, rheumatoid arthritis, and other inflammatory disorders.

• Stimulation of Gastric Juices: Cayenne pepper, through capsaicin, is believed to stimulate saliva production, gastric juices, and enzymes, aiding digestion and relieving indigestion, gas, and bloating.

• Metabolism Booster: Capsaicin is thought to increase metabolism temporarily, leading to increased calorie burning and potentially aiding weight management efforts. It may also reduce appetite.

• Improvement of Circulation: Capsaicin's vasodilatory effect may improve blood circulation and reduce the risk of blood clots. It could potentially lower cholesterol levels, supporting heart health.

• Congestion Relief: Cayenne pepper's ability to stimulate secretions and clear nasal passages can offer relief from congestion, making it beneficial for colds, sinus congestion, or sore throats.

• Free Radical Scavenging: Cayenne pepper contains antioxidants like carotenoids and flavonoids that help neutralize free radicals, reducing oxidative stress and supporting overall health.

• Anticancer Properties: Emerging research suggests that capsaicin may have the potential to inhibit the growth of certain cancer cells. However, more studies are needed to confirm its effectiveness.

• Topical Pain Relief: When applied topically, capsaicin-based creams or ointments can offer localized pain relief for sore muscles, joint pain, or nerve-related pain.

• Potential for Wound Healing: Cayenne pepper's antibacterial properties, attributed to capsaicin, may assist in preventing infection and promoting wound healing when applied topically.

These properties highlight the diverse therapeutic potential of cayenne pepper, particularly attributed to its active component, capsaicin. However, individual responses may vary, and it's advisable to use cayenne pepper-based remedies with caution, especially if you have specific health concerns or are sensitive to spicy foods. Consulting with a healthcare professional is recommended before using cayenne pepper for medicinal purposes.

## THE DIVERSE HEALTH BENEFITS OF CAYENNE PEPPER

Cayenne pepper offers diverse health benefits attributed to its active compound, capsaicin, and other components. Here's a detailed overview of its roles in various aspects of health:

• Capsaicin's Analgesic Effect: Capsaicin interacts with pain receptors, reducing the perception of pain. Topical applications of capsaicin-based creams or patches offer relief from muscle pain, joint pain (arthritis), neuropathic pain, and headaches by desensitizing nerves.

• Stimulation of Digestive Processes: Capsaicin in cayenne pepper stimulates saliva and gastric juices, aiding digestion. It can alleviate indigestion, gas, and bloating by promoting the release of digestive enzymes.

• Vasodilatory Effects: Cayenne pepper's capsaicin may promote better blood circulation by widening blood vessels.

Improved circulation supports heart health and may reduce the risk of blood clots.

• Increased Metabolism: Capsaicin temporarily boosts metabolism, leading to increased calorie burning and potential support for weight management efforts. It may also reduce appetite, aiding in calorie control.

• Cholesterol Regulation: Capsaicin may help lower cholesterol levels and improve heart health by reducing bad cholesterol (LDL) and increasing good cholesterol (HDL).

• Congestion Relief: Cayenne pepper's ability to stimulate secretions aids in clearing nasal passages, providing relief from congestion due to colds or sinus issues.

• Reduction of Oxidative Stress: Cayenne pepper contains antioxidants that help neutralize free radicals, reducing oxidative stress and supporting overall health.

• Reduction of Inflammation: Capsaicin exhibits anti-inflammatory properties, assisting in reducing inflammation associated with conditions like osteoarthritis and rheumatoid arthritis.

• Appetite Suppression: Capsaicin may help reduce appetite, potentially aiding in weight management by promoting satiety and reducing overall calorie intake.

• Enhanced Digestion: Cayenne pepper's ability to stimulate gastric juices and enzymes may aid digestion, improving overall digestive health and alleviating digestive discomfort.

These diverse health benefits demonstrate the multifaceted role of cayenne pepper, primarily due to the presence of capsaicin and other bioactive compounds. However, individual responses to cayenne pepper can vary, and caution should be exercised, especially if considering its use for specific health concerns. Consulting with a healthcare professional is recommended for personalized advice.

# CHAPTER TWO



Cayenne pepper, known for its spicy heat and diverse culinary and medicinal uses, includes various types or varieties, each with unique characteristics in terms of flavor, heat level, and appearance. Some of the different types of cayenne pepper include:

• Cayenne Pepper (Capsicum annuum): This is the general term used to refer to the hot chili peppers belonging to the Capsicum annuum species. Different cultivars and varieties within this species can exhibit variations in size, shape, color, and heat intensity.

• Long Red Cayenne: These are elongated, slender peppers with a bright red color when ripe. They typically grow to about 6 to 8 inches long and are known for their medium to high heat level.

• Ring of Fire Cayenne: This variety is similar to the long red cayenne but is known for its hotter and more intense spiciness. It is often used in hot sauces and spicy dishes.

• Thai Cayenne: Smaller and slimmer than traditional cayenne peppers, Thai cayenne peppers pack a significant amount of heat. They're commonly used in Thai cuisine for their intense spiciness.

• African Bird's Eye Cayenne: Also known as peri-peri or piri-piri peppers, these small, fiery peppers are widely used in African and Portuguese cuisines. They are extremely hot and are often used to make hot sauces.

• Purple Cayenne: These cayenne peppers ripen to a purple color before turning red. They offer a slightly milder heat compared to some other cayenne varieties.

• Golden Cayenne: This variety, as the name suggests, ripens to a bright yellow or golden color instead of the traditional red. The heat level is similar to the red cayenne pepper.

• Demon Red Cayenne: Known for its intense heat, the Demon Red cayenne pepper is fiery and offers a high level of spiciness, making it suitable for those who enjoy extremely hot peppers.

Each type of cayenne pepper varies in terms of heat, flavor, and appearance, providing options for culinary use based on personal preferences and the desired level of spiciness in dishes. Whether you prefer a milder heat or seek out the intense fiery flavor, cayenne pepper varieties offer a range of choices for different culinary creations.

## THE USES AND PROPERTIES OF THE DIFFERENT TYPES OF CAYENNE PEPPER

The different types of cayenne peppers possess varying heat levels, flavors, and characteristics, offering diverse uses in culinary dishes and herbal remedies. Here's a breakdown of the uses and properties of some common types of cayenne pepper:

Long Red Cayenne:

• Heat Level: Medium to high heat.

• Uses: Widely used in cooking to add heat and flavor to dishes such as sauces, salsas, marinades, and pickles. It's also suitable for drying and grinding into cayenne powder for seasoning.

Ring of Fire Cayenne:

• Heat Level: Higher than the traditional long red cayenne.

• Uses: Ideal for adding intense heat to hot sauces, spicy dishes, and recipes that require a higher level of spiciness. Can also be dried and ground for cayenne powder.

## Thai Cayenne:

• Heat Level: Intense and very spicy.

• Uses: Commonly used in Thai cuisine for its fiery heat. Adds heat to soups, stir-fries, curries, and spicy dips.

## African Bird's Eye Cayenne (Peri-Peri):

• Heat Level: Extremely hot.

• Uses: Frequently used to make hot sauces, marinades, and seasoning blends. Its intense heat is popular in African and Portuguese cuisines for adding fiery flavor to dishes.

## Purple Cayenne:

• Heat Level: Moderate heat.

• Uses: Adds color and mild to moderate heat to dishes, similar to traditional cayenne pepper. Can be used in sauces, pickling, or as a colorful garnish.

Golden Cayenne:

• Heat Level: Similar to the red cayenne pepper.

• Uses: Offers a visual variation in dishes, providing a bright yellow or golden color. Used similarly to traditional cayenne pepper for seasoning and spicing up recipes.

Demon Red Cayenne:

• Heat Level: Extremely high heat.

• Uses: Ideal for those who enjoy exceptionally spicy food. Used sparingly due to its intense heat, added to dishes where extreme spiciness is desired.

Each type of cayenne pepper, with its unique heat level and flavor profile, can be employed to customize the spiciness and taste of various dishes. Additionally, these peppers can be dried and ground into powder form for use as a seasoning or incorporated into herbal remedies, depending on the desired heat intensity and flavor. When using these peppers in recipes or remedies, it's important to consider their heat levels and adjust quantities based on personal preferences and tolerance for spiciness.

# DIFFERENT WAYS TO INCORPORATE CAYENNE PEPPER INTO REMEDIES

Cayenne pepper, with its active component capsaicin and other beneficial compounds, can be incorporated into remedies in various ways for its potential health benefits. Here are different methods to utilize cayenne pepper in remedies:

• Capsaicin Creams or Ointments: Mix cayenne powder with a carrier oil (like coconut oil or olive oil) to create a paste. Apply the paste topically to areas experiencing pain, such as sore muscles or joints, for its analgesic properties.

• Cayenne Capsules: Encapsulate cayenne powder or use commercially available cayenne supplements. These can be taken orally for digestive support, metabolism boosting, or as part of a detox regimen.

• Cayenne Infusion: Mix a small amount of cayenne pepper powder with warm water and lemon juice to create a digestive tonic. This mixture may aid digestion and relieve indigestion.

• Cayenne Herbal Tea: Infuse cayenne pepper in hot water along with other herbs like ginger or peppermint for a soothing tea. It can help with congestion, circulation, and digestion.

• Cayenne Tincture: Prepare a tincture using cayenne pepper and alcohol (like vodka). The tincture can be used in small amounts for digestive support or to alleviate sore throat when diluted in water.

• Cayenne Detox Beverages: Combine cayenne pepper with other detoxifying ingredients like lemon juice, apple cider vinegar, and water for a cleansing drink. It may aid in detoxification and metabolism.

• Cayenne Poultice: Create a poultice using cayenne powder mixed with water or oil, then apply it to areas of the body experiencing pain or inflammation. This method may help with localized pain relief.

• Capsaicin-based Salves: Mix cayenne powder with beeswax and a carrier oil (like coconut oil) to create a homemade salve or balm. This can be used topically for pain relief or muscle soreness.

• Incorporate in Food: Use cayenne pepper in cooking to add flavor and spice to various dishes, soups, sauces, or marinades. It can be used in both savory and sweet recipes to add heat.

• Capsaicin Nasal Spray: Dilute a small amount of cayenne powder in saline solution to create a nasal spray. It may help clear nasal congestion when used in small quantities.

Remember, when incorporating cayenne pepper into remedies, it's essential to start with small amounts and consider individual tolerance levels, especially concerning spiciness. Additionally, consulting with a healthcare professional or herbalist before using cayenne pepper for specific health concerns is advisable, especially if you have underlying health conditions or sensitivities.

## APPLICATION OF CAYENNE PEPPER

Cayenne pepper, known for its spicy flavor and potential health benefits due to its active component capsaicin, has various applications in cooking, herbal remedies, and even some household uses. Here are several ways cayenne pepper can be applied:

• Cooking Spice: Use as a spice to add heat and flavor to a wide range of dishes such as soups, stews, curries, sauces, marinades, and meat rubs.

• Condiment: Create homemade hot sauces, salsas, and dips by combining cayenne pepper with other ingredients like vinegar, tomatoes, onions, and garlic.

• Seasoning: Sprinkle on roasted vegetables, popcorn, eggs, or pasta dishes to enhance flavor and add a spicy kick.

## Herbal Remedies:

• Pain Relief: Prepare capsaicin-based creams or ointments for topical application to alleviate muscle pain, arthritis, and neuropathic pain.

• Digestive Aid: Mix cayenne pepper with warm water and lemon for a digestive tonic to help with indigestion and promote better digestion.

• Detoxification: Combine cayenne pepper with other detoxifying ingredients like lemon juice and apple cider vinegar for cleansing drinks or detox regimens.

• Topical Applications: Use cayenne pepper poultices or compresses topically for pain relief or to stimulate circulation in specific areas.

Household Uses:

• Pest Deterrent: Create a natural deterrent for certain pests like insects or squirrels by sprinkling cayenne pepper around gardens or areas where pests frequent.

• Bird Repellent: Dust cayenne pepper around bird feeders or garden plants to deter birds from eating seeds or fruits.

• Ant Repellent: Use cayenne pepper near entry points to repel ants. The spicy scent can deter them from entering the house.

• Cleansing Agent: Incorporate cayenne pepper into homemade cleaning solutions as a natural disinfectant or to help break down grease on surfaces.

When using cayenne pepper, it's essential to be mindful of its heat level, especially for individuals sensitive to spicy foods. Additionally, start with small amounts and gradually increase to suit personal preferences. If using cayenne pepper for medicinal purposes, consult with a healthcare professional for guidance on appropriate dosages and applications.

## CAYENNE PEPPER AND PAIN RELIEF

Cayenne pepper, specifically its active component capsaicin, is associated with pain relief due to its interaction with sensory nerves and modulation of pain perception. Here's a detailed discussion on cayenne pepper and its role in pain relief:

Mechanism of Action:

*Interaction with Nerves:*

• Capsaicin interacts with a specific receptor in nerve endings known as the Transient Receptor Potential Vanilloid 1 (TRPV1) receptor.

• TRPV1 receptors are involved in the transmission of pain signals to the brain. Capsaicin binds to these receptors, leading to the initial perception of heat or a burning sensation.

*Desensitization Effect:*

• Prolonged or repeated exposure to capsaicin leads to a reduction in the sensitivity of TRPV1 receptors. This desensitization results in decreased pain perception over time.

Pain Relief Applications:

*Topical Capsaicin Products:*

• Capsaicin-based creams, gels, or patches are commonly used topically for pain relief.

• These products are applied directly to the skin over the affected area, such as sore muscles, joint pain (e.g., arthritis), or neuropathic pain.

*Efficacy in Various Types of Pain:*

• Muscle Pain: Topical capsaicin has shown efficacy in providing relief from muscle soreness and stiffness by desensitizing pain receptors.

• Arthritis: Studies indicate that capsaicin can help alleviate pain associated with osteoarthritis and rheumatoid arthritis when used topically.

• Neuropathic Pain: Capsaicin creams have been found to be beneficial in managing certain types of neuropathic pain, such as diabetic neuropathy.

Evidence Supporting Pain Relief:

*Clinical Studies:*

• Research studies have demonstrated the effectiveness of capsaicin in managing various types of pain.

• A study published in the "Journal of Clinical Pharmacy and Therapeutics" showed that capsaicin patches provided relief from painful diabetic peripheral neuropathy.

• Another study in "Pain Medicine" found that capsaicin cream significantly reduced pain associated with osteoarthritis compared to a placebo.

*Pain Reduction Over Time:*

• While the immediate application of capsaicin might cause an initial burning sensation, consistent use can lead to diminished pain perception as the nerve endings become desensitized.

• Individual Tolerance: Sensitivity to capsaicin varies among individuals. Some people may experience discomfort or a burning sensation initially, while others may tolerate it better.

• Application Frequency: It's recommended to follow the instructions provided with capsaicin-based products, gradually increasing the application frequency to prevent skin irritation.

• Consultation with Healthcare Professionals: Individuals with sensitive skin, allergies, or specific health conditions should consult healthcare providers before using capsaicin-based products for pain relief.

While capsaicin in cayenne pepper offers potential benefits for pain relief, its effectiveness can vary from person to person. It's essential to use these products cautiously, follow usage guidelines, and seek advice from healthcare professionals for personalized recommendations.

Cayenne pepper has been associated with potential benefits for digestive health due to its active compound, capsaicin, and other bioactive components. Here's a detailed discussion on cayenne pepper and its role in digestive health:

Effects on Digestion:

• Stimulation of Digestive Processes: Cayenne pepper is believed to stimulate saliva production and gastric juices, promoting better digestion. Capsaicin in cayenne pepper may trigger the release of digestive enzymes, aiding in the breakdown of food in the stomach.

• Relief from Indigestion: Some anecdotal evidence suggests that consuming cayenne pepper might help alleviate symptoms of indigestion by improving digestive function.

• Enhancement of Metabolism: Capsaicin has been associated with a transient increase in metabolism. This increase in metabolic rate could potentially aid in the digestion and breakdown of food.

Scientific Evidence and Studies:

• Limited Specific Studies: There is a lack of direct scientific evidence specifically focused on cayenne pepper's effects on digestive health. Most research on capsaicin's effects on digestion is conducted using purified capsaicin supplements or extracts.

• Capsaicin and Gastric Mucosal Blood Flow: Some studies suggest that capsaicin may stimulate gastric mucosal blood flow, potentially aiding in maintaining a healthy stomach lining. However, the application of this evidence specifically to cayenne pepper itself requires further research.

Considerations and Precautions:

• Individual Tolerance and Sensitivity: Cayenne pepper's spiciness might not be well-tolerated by everyone, especially individuals with sensitive stomachs or gastrointestinal conditions. Some individuals might experience heartburn, irritation, or exacerbation of existing digestive issues due to cayenne's heat.

• Moderation and Dosage: Using cayenne pepper in moderation and gradually increasing its intake may help individuals gauge their tolerance levels. Excessive consumption of cayenne pepper may lead to irritation or discomfort in the digestive tract.

## Application Methods:

• Ingestion in Foods: Cayenne pepper can be incorporated into various dishes, including soups, stews, sauces, and marinades, to add flavor and potentially stimulate digestion.

• Digestive Tonic: Mixing a small amount of cayenne pepper with warm water and lemon juice is believed to create a digestive tonic that may help alleviate digestive discomfort.

## Precautions and Consultation:

• Consultation with Healthcare Providers: Individuals with gastrointestinal conditions like acid reflux, ulcers, or irritable bowel syndrome (IBS) should consult healthcare providers before using cayenne pepper for digestive purposes.

• Observation and Personalized Approach: Individuals should observe their own reactions to cayenne pepper and consider their own tolerance levels, adjusting consumption accordingly.

While cayenne pepper might have potential benefits for digestive health based on anecdotal evidence and its active compound, more comprehensive scientific studies specifically on cayenne pepper are needed to firmly establish its effects on digestive processes and overall gastrointestinal health. As with any dietary change or addition, moderation and individual considerations are crucial. Consulting a healthcare professional is recommended, especially for those with existing digestive issues or concerns.

## CAYENNE PEPPER AND WEIGHT MANAGEMENT

Cayenne pepper, containing the active compound capsaicin, has been associated with potential benefits for weight management and weight loss due to its effects on metabolism, appetite regulation, and fat oxidation. Here's a detailed discussion on cayenne pepper and its role in weight management:

Effects on Metabolism and Fat Burning:

• Increase in Metabolic Rate: Capsaicin has been found to temporarily increase thermogenesis, raising the body's temperature and boosting metabolic activity. This increase in metabolism can lead to greater calorie expenditure.

• Enhanced Fat Oxidation: Capsaicin may promote the oxidation of fats, potentially aiding in the breakdown of stored fats for energy, contributing to weight loss efforts.

## Appetite Regulation and Reduced Caloric Intake:

• Appetite Suppression: Capsaicin may help suppress appetite by promoting a feeling of fullness or satiety, potentially reducing overall calorie intake. Some studies suggest that capsaicin intake may lead to a decrease in food cravings and subsequent calorie consumption.

• Impact on Ghrelin Levels: Ghrelin is a hormone that stimulates hunger. Some research suggests that capsaicin might influence ghrelin levels, possibly reducing hunger sensations.

## Scientific Evidence and Studies:

### *Metabolic Effects:*

• A study published in the "International Journal of Obesity" reported that capsaicin supplementation increased energy expenditure and fat oxidation in participants.

• Another study in the "American Journal of Clinical Nutrition" showed that capsaicin intake moderately increased energy expenditure.

*Appetite Suppression:*

• Research published in "Appetite" demonstrated that capsaicinoids might reduce hunger and increase satiety, potentially aiding in weight management.

Considerations and Precautions:

• Individual Responses: Responses to cayenne pepper and capsaicin can vary among individuals. Some may experience a greater impact on metabolism and appetite suppression, while others may have a more modest response.

• Gradual Increase and Tolerance: Starting with small amounts of cayenne pepper and gradually increasing intake might help individuals gauge their tolerance levels.

Application Methods:

• Incorporation in Foods: Adding cayenne pepper to various recipes, such as soups, stir-fries, or seasoning blends, can introduce its thermogenic properties and potentially aid in weight management.

• Capsaicin Supplements: Some individuals opt for capsaicin supplements to support weight loss efforts. However, it's crucial to consult healthcare providers before taking supplements.

Precautions and Consultation:

• Health Conditions and Medications: Individuals with gastrointestinal conditions, allergies, or using certain medications should consult healthcare providers before using cayenne pepper or capsaicin for weight management.

• Lifestyle Factors: Cayenne pepper should be considered as a part of a comprehensive weight management plan that includes a balanced diet and regular physical activity.

While cayenne pepper and capsaicin may offer potential benefits for weight management, they should not be seen as standalone solutions for weight loss. Integrating cayenne pepper into a balanced diet and healthy lifestyle, along with consulting healthcare providers, can contribute to overall weight management goals. Individual responses may vary, and caution should be exercised, especially by those with specific health conditions or sensitivities.

## CAYENNE PEPPER AND COLD AND FLU RELIEF

Cayenne pepper, particularly its active component capsaicin, has been associated with potential benefits for alleviating symptoms of colds and flu, mainly due to its ability to provide relief from congestion and its potential immune-boosting properties. Here's a detailed discussion on cayenne pepper and its role in cold and flu relief:

Effects on Congestion Relief:

• Nasal Decongestion: Capsaicin can help clear nasal passages by thinning mucus and facilitating its expulsion. It works by stimulating the release of watery secretions, aiding in decongestion.

• Sinus Relief: The heat from cayenne pepper may help open up sinus passages and relieve pressure, providing relief from sinus congestion associated with colds and flu.

Immune-Boosting Properties:

*Antibacterial and Antiviral Properties:*

• While direct evidence specific to cayenne pepper is limited, capsaicin has shown some antibacterial and antiviral properties in laboratory studies.

• These properties might potentially aid in combating viral and bacterial infections, contributing to overall immune function.

Scientific Evidence and Studies:

• Nasal Congestion Relief: A study published in the "Annals of Allergy, Asthma & Immunology" suggested that capsaicin nasal spray provided relief from nonallergic rhinitis symptoms by improving nasal airflow.

• Antibacterial and Antiviral Effects: Research in the "Journal of Ethnopharmacology" suggested that capsaicin exhibits potential antiviral effects against certain viruses. Additionally, a study in "PLoS ONE" showed that capsaicin had antibacterial properties against certain bacteria.

Considerations and Precautions:

• Individual Tolerance: Cayenne pepper's spiciness may not be well-tolerated by everyone, especially those with sensitive nasal passages or skin. It's important to start with small amounts and gauge individual tolerance levels.

• Potential Irritation: Direct contact with mucous membranes or sensitive areas can cause irritation or discomfort. Avoid applying cayenne pepper directly to sensitive skin without proper dilution.

Application Methods:

• Nasal Rinse or Spray: Diluted cayenne pepper mixed with saline solution can be used as a homemade nasal rinse or spray to alleviate nasal congestion. Caution should be exercised to ensure the solution is appropriately diluted to prevent irritation.

• Incorporation in Foods: Adding cayenne pepper to soups or hot beverages might offer temporary relief from cold and flu symptoms by promoting nasal decongestion.

• Health Conditions and Sensitivities: Individuals with allergies, respiratory conditions (e.g., asthma), or sensitive nasal passages should consult healthcare providers before using cayenne pepper for cold and flu relief.

• Complementary Approach: Cayenne pepper can be considered as a complementary approach to alleviate symptoms, but it should not replace conventional treatments or medical advice.

While cayenne pepper might offer relief from certain symptoms associated with colds and flu, its effectiveness can vary among individuals. It should be used cautiously, especially by those with sensitivities or underlying health conditions. Consulting healthcare providers for personalized guidance is recommended before using cayenne pepper for cold and flu relief.

# CAYENNE PEPPER AND ANTI-INFLAMMATORY PROPERTIES

Cayenne pepper, containing the active compound capsaicin, has been studied for its potential anti-inflammatory properties, which may aid in reducing inflammation and related discomfort. Here's a detailed discussion on cayenne pepper and its role in providing anti-inflammatory effects:

## Mechanism of Anti-Inflammatory Action:

• Interaction with TRPV1 Receptors: Capsaicin interacts with Transient Receptor Potential Vanilloid 1 (TRPV1) receptors in the body. TRPV1 receptors are involved in the perception of pain and the regulation of inflammatory responses.

• Modulation of Inflammatory Responses: Capsaicin's interaction with TRPV1 receptors can modulate the release of certain neurotransmitters involved in inflammation, potentially reducing inflammation and associated pain.

## Effects on Inflammation:

• Pain Reduction: By acting on TRPV1 receptors, capsaicin may help alleviate pain associated with inflammatory conditions like osteoarthritis and rheumatoid arthritis.

• Potential Reduction in Inflammatory Markers: Some studies suggest that capsaicin might decrease the production or release of certain inflammatory markers, contributing to anti-inflammatory effects.

Scientific Evidence and Studies:

*Studies on Inflammatory Conditions:*

• A study published in the "Journal of Clinical Investigation" suggested that capsaicin might have anti-inflammatory effects by modulating immune cell functions.

• Another study in the "Journal of Pain Research" reported that capsaicin-based topical creams showed promise in reducing inflammation-related pain.

*Effects on Inflammatory Markers:*

• Research published in "PLOS ONE" indicated that capsaicin may suppress the production of inflammatory cytokines in certain cell cultures, potentially reducing inflammation.

Considerations and Precautions:

• Individual Responses: Responses to cayenne pepper and capsaicin can vary among individuals. Some people may experience more significant relief from inflammation than others.

• Potential Sensitivities: Cayenne pepper's spiciness might not be well-tolerated by everyone, especially individuals with sensitive skin or mucous membranes.

## Application Methods:

• Topical Application: Capsaicin-based creams or ointments can be applied topically to areas experiencing inflammation, such as joints affected by arthritis. These topical preparations are believed to reduce pain and inflammation in localized areas.

## Precautions and Consultation:

• Health Conditions and Medications: Individuals with skin sensitivities, allergies, or those using certain medications should consult healthcare providers before using capsaicin-based products for anti-inflammatory purposes.

• Complementary Approach: Cayenne pepper can be considered as a complementary approach to help alleviate inflammation and associated discomfort but should not replace conventional medical treatments.

While cayenne pepper, particularly capsaicin, shows promise in providing anti-inflammatory effects, more comprehensive research is needed to confirm its efficacy in managing inflammatory conditions. It's essential to use capsaicin-based products cautiously, especially by those with sensitivities or specific health concerns. Consulting healthcare providers before using cayenne pepper for anti-inflammatory purposes is advisable for personalized guidance.

## CAYENNE PEPPER AND ANTI-FUNGAL PROPERTIES

Cayenne pepper, particularly its active compound capsaicin, has demonstrated some potential as an antifungal agent against certain fungal species. Here's a detailed discussion on cayenne pepper and its role in possessing anti-fungal properties:

Antifungal Mechanism of Action:

• Fungal Growth Inhibition: Capsaicin in cayenne pepper has shown the ability to inhibit the growth and spread of certain fungal species. It interferes with the fungal cell wall and disrupts their membrane integrity, hindering their ability to thrive and reproduce.

• Disruption of Fungal Biofilms: Capsaicin has demonstrated the potential to disrupt fungal biofilms, which are colonies of fungi protected by a matrix that makes them resistant to antifungal agents.

## Effects on Fungal Species:

• Antifungal Activity: Research studies have shown that capsaicin exhibits varying degrees of antifungal activity against fungal strains such as Candida albicans, Aspergillus spp., and dermatophytes.

## Scientific Evidence and Studies:

• In vitro Studies: Studies published in journals like "Mycoses" and "Journal of Applied Microbiology" have demonstrated capsaicin's inhibitory effects on fungal growth in laboratory settings. These studies suggest capsaicin's potential as an antifungal agent, particularly against Candida species and certain dermatophytes.

## Considerations and Precautions:

• Varied Efficacy: The effectiveness of capsaicin against fungal strains may vary. Some fungal species might be more susceptible to its antifungal properties than others.

- Concentration and Application: The concentration of capsaicin and the mode of application might affect its efficacy as an antifungal agent. Topical applications may be more relevant for localized fungal infections.

Application Methods:

- Topical Use: Capsaicin-based creams or ointments could potentially be applied topically to areas affected by certain fungal infections, though further research is needed to establish its efficacy.

- Incorporation in Formulations: Capsaicin could potentially be incorporated into antifungal formulations or combined with other natural antifungal agents for increased efficacy.

Precautions and Consultation:

- Skin Sensitivities and Allergies: Individuals with sensitive skin or allergies to capsaicin should use caution when considering cayenne pepper for antifungal purposes.

- Consultation with Healthcare Providers: It's advisable to consult healthcare providers or dermatologists before using capsaicin-based products for antifungal purposes, especially for persistent or severe fungal infections.

While cayenne pepper, particularly capsaicin, has shown promise in laboratory studies as an antifungal agent, further research is necessary to establish its effectiveness and safety for treating fungal infections in humans. It should be considered as a potential complementary approach alongside conventional antifungal treatments, especially under the guidance of healthcare providers. Individual responses and the specific fungal strains need to be considered when utilizing capsaicin for its antifungal properties.

## CAYENNE PEPPER AND DETOXIFICATION

Cayenne pepper is often associated with detoxification due to its potential ability to stimulate various bodily functions, aid digestion, and support metabolic processes. Here's a detailed discussion on cayenne pepper and its purported role in detoxification:

Effects on Detoxification:

• Metabolism Boost: Capsaicin, the active compound in cayenne pepper, is believed to temporarily increase metabolic rate, potentially aiding in the breakdown of toxins stored in fat cells.

• Promotion of Digestive Processes: Cayenne pepper is thought to stimulate saliva production and gastric juices, enhancing digestion and the elimination of waste from the body.

• Circulation Improvement: The heat generated by capsaicin in cayenne pepper may help improve blood circulation. Improved circulation could potentially aid in toxin removal by enhancing organ function.

Effects on Digestion and Elimination:

• Supports Bowel Movements: Cayenne pepper's potential to stimulate digestion and bowel movements might aid in the elimination of waste and toxins from the body.

• Antibacterial Properties: Some research suggests capsaicin may possess antibacterial properties, which might indirectly support gut health and detoxification by reducing harmful bacterial overgrowth.

• Limited Direct Studies: While cayenne pepper is often included in detox regimens, there is a lack of direct scientific evidence specifically focusing on its role in detoxification.

• General Health Benefits: Studies have shown some health benefits associated with capsaicin, such as improved metabolism and circulation, which are indirectly related to detoxification.

Considerations and Precautions:

• Comprehensive Approach: Detoxification should be approached comprehensively, considering a balanced diet, hydration, exercise, and overall lifestyle modifications rather than relying solely on cayenne pepper.

• Individual Responses: Responses to detoxification methods, including cayenne pepper, can vary among individuals. Factors such as health status and metabolism play a role in its effectiveness.

Application Methods:

• Detox Drinks: Some detoxification regimens include cayenne pepper in cleansing drinks or tonics combined with lemon juice, water, and other detoxifying ingredients.

• Incorporation in Foods: Adding cayenne pepper to foods as a seasoning can be a way to introduce its potential detoxifying properties into the diet.

Precautions and Consultation:

• Health Conditions and Medications: Individuals with gastrointestinal conditions, allergies, or those taking specific medications should consult healthcare providers before incorporating cayenne pepper into a detoxification regimen.

• Gradual Introduction: Gradually introducing cayenne pepper into the diet or detox regimen may help individuals gauge their tolerance levels and reduce the risk of adverse reactions.

While cayenne pepper is often promoted as a component of detox regimens due to its potential to support digestion and metabolism, there is limited direct scientific evidence specifically addressing its role in detoxification. It should be used cautiously and as part of a holistic approach to health and wellness. Consulting healthcare providers or nutritionists before starting any detoxification program involving cayenne pepper is advisable, especially for individuals with underlying health conditions or sensitivities.

## CAYENNE PEPPER AND MIGRAINE RELIEF

Cayenne pepper, particularly its active component capsaicin, has been studied for its potential in migraine relief. While its mechanism of action isn't entirely clear, capsaicin's interaction with pain pathways and its effects on blood vessels are believed to play a role in alleviating migraine symptoms. Here's a detailed discussion on cayenne pepper and its role in migraine relief:

Effects on Migraine Relief:

• Pain Relief: Capsaicin has shown potential in blocking Substance P, a neurotransmitter involved in pain transmission. This action may help reduce pain sensitivity associated with migraines.

- Vasodilation and Vasoconstriction: Capsaicin can cause initial vasodilation (expansion of blood vessels) followed by vasoconstriction (narrowing of blood vessels), potentially aiding in migraine relief by modulating blood flow.

## Scientific Evidence and Studies:

- Limited Direct Studies: Research specifically focusing on cayenne pepper's effects on migraines is limited. Some studies have investigated capsaicin's role in headache disorders, but further research is needed to draw definitive conclusions regarding its efficacy for migraines.

- Capsaicin Nasal Spray: A nasal spray containing capsaicin has been studied for cluster headaches and migraines. Some research suggests it may provide relief, though more robust studies are necessary.

## Considerations and Precautions:

- Individual Responses: Responses to cayenne pepper or capsaicin-based treatments for migraines can vary among individuals. Some may find relief, while others might experience irritation or worsening of symptoms.

• Potential Skin Irritation: Direct contact with capsaicin may cause skin irritation or a burning sensation. Using capsaicin-based products cautiously is important, especially around sensitive areas.

Application Methods:

• Capsaicin-Based Creams or Ointments: Some individuals apply capsaicin-based creams topically to the forehead or temples to potentially alleviate migraine pain. However, caution is advised due to potential skin irritation.

• Nasal Sprays or Solutions: Capsaicin nasal sprays or solutions are used in some studies for cluster headaches or migraines. These are administered with caution due to the potential for nasal irritation.

Precautions and Consultation:

• Consultation with Healthcare Providers: Individuals with migraines or chronic headaches should consult healthcare providers before using capsaicin-based products for migraine relief, especially if using other medications or treatments.

• Complementary Approach: Cayenne pepper or capsaicin-based treatments should be considered as a complementary approach to managing migraines and should not replace prescribed migraine medications without medical advice.

While cayenne pepper, specifically capsaicin, has shown some potential in migraine relief based on preliminary studies and its effects on pain pathways and blood vessels, more comprehensive and robust research is needed to establish its efficacy and safety for managing migraines. It's advisable for individuals with migraines to consult healthcare providers for personalized guidance before using cayenne pepper or capsaicin-based treatments as part of their migraine management plan.

## CAYENNE PEPPER AND IMPROVED BLOOD CIRCULATION

Cayenne pepper, containing the active compound capsaicin, has been associated with potential benefits for blood circulation due to its ability to stimulate circulation and improve blood flow. Here's a detailed discussion on cayenne pepper and its role in enhancing blood circulation:

• Vasodilation: Capsaicin, when consumed, can cause a temporary dilation of blood vessels. This vasodilatory effect widens the blood vessels, promoting increased blood flow throughout the body.

• Improved Peripheral Circulation: Cayenne pepper may particularly benefit peripheral circulation by enhancing blood flow to the extremities, potentially aiding in warming cold hands or feet.

Scientific Evidence and Studies:

• Capsaicin's Vasodilatory Effects: Research published in the journal "Pharmacological Reviews" suggests that capsaicin induces vasodilation by affecting sensory nerves and leading to the release of vasodilatory substances.

• Blood Flow Improvement: A study in "The American Journal of Clinical Nutrition" indicated that capsaicin increased blood flow in healthy adults following its consumption.

Cardiovascular Benefits:

• Heart Health Support: Improved circulation can benefit heart health by ensuring better delivery of oxygen and nutrients to the heart and other organs.

• Blood Pressure Regulation: Some studies suggest that capsaicin may help regulate blood pressure by influencing blood vessel tone, though more research is needed in this area.

Considerations and Precautions:

• Individual Responses: Responses to cayenne pepper's effects on blood circulation can vary among individuals. Some people might experience a more noticeable increase in blood flow than others.

• Potential Sensitivities: Cayenne pepper's spiciness might not be well-tolerated by everyone, especially individuals with gastrointestinal conditions or sensitive stomachs.

Application Methods:

• Consumption in Foods: Incorporating cayenne pepper into the diet by adding it to dishes or consuming it in beverages might provide the vasodilatory benefits associated with improved circulation.

• Topical Use: Some individuals use capsaicin-based creams or ointments topically on specific areas to potentially improve local blood flow.



• Health Conditions and Medications: Individuals with specific health conditions (like bleeding disorders) or those using medications affecting blood clotting should consult healthcare providers before using cayenne pepper for improved circulation.

• Gradual Introduction: Gradually introducing cayenne pepper into the diet may help individuals gauge their tolerance levels and minimize potential gastrointestinal irritation.

While cayenne pepper, specifically capsaicin, has shown promise in improving blood circulation based on its vasodilatory effects, more comprehensive studies are needed to confirm its efficacy and safety in promoting circulation. It should be used cautiously, especially by individuals with specific health conditions or sensitivities. Consulting healthcare providers for personalized guidance before using cayenne pepper for improving blood circulation is advisable, particularly for those with underlying health concerns.

## DOSAGE RECOMMENDATIONS BASED ON THE SPECIFIC REMEDY AND INDIVIDUAL FACTORS

Dosage recommendations for cayenne pepper or capsaicin-based remedies can vary significantly based on the specific remedy, individual factors such as age, health status, and sensitivity to capsaicin. Here are some general guidelines for common forms of cayenne pepper remedies and factors to consider:

### Capsaicin Creams or Topical Applications:

• General Dosage: Follow the manufacturer's instructions or as advised by a healthcare professional.

• Initial Application: Start with a small amount on a small area of skin to test for sensitivity or allergic reactions.

• Frequency: Typically applied 3 to 4 times daily to the affected area.

• Gradual Increase: If well-tolerated, the frequency or amount can be gradually increased.

## Oral Consumption or Capsules:

• Powdered Cayenne Pepper: Start with a small amount, around 1/4 to 1/2 teaspoon, mixed with food or beverages. Gradually increase the amount based on tolerance.

• Capsules or Supplements: Dosage can vary widely based on the concentration of capsaicin. Follow the instructions on the product label or as directed by a healthcare provider.

## Detox Drinks or Cleanses:

• Detox Drink with Cayenne Pepper: Recipes may vary but usually include a small amount of cayenne pepper mixed with water, lemon juice, and other detoxifying ingredients. Start with small amounts and adjust according to personal tolerance.

## Factors to Consider:

• Individual Sensitivity: Some individuals are more sensitive to capsaicin and may experience gastrointestinal discomfort or skin irritation. Start with smaller doses to assess tolerance.

• Health Conditions: People with gastrointestinal issues, allergies, or certain medical conditions may need to avoid or limit cayenne pepper intake. Consulting a healthcare professional is advisable.

• Age and Weight: Dosage might need adjustment based on age and body weight. Children and older adults might require smaller amounts.

• Medication Interactions: Capsaicin might interact with certain medications. Those taking blood thinners or medications for heart conditions should consult healthcare providers before using capsaicin-based remedies.

• Gradual Introduction: Whether topically or orally, gradually introducing cayenne pepper allows individuals to gauge their tolerance and minimize adverse reactions.

• Specific Remedies: Different remedies, such as pain relief creams versus detox drinks, might require different dosages. Always follow specific guidelines for each remedy.

It's crucial to emphasize that these dosage recommendations are general guidelines, and personalized advice from a healthcare professional should be sought before starting any new cayenne pepper-based remedy, especially for those with underlying health conditions or concerns.

# CHAPTER THREE

## THE IMPORTANCE OF MODERATION

Moderation is crucial when using cayenne pepper or capsaicin-based remedies due to its potent and potentially intense effects on the body. Here are the key reasons highlighting the importance of moderation:

• Gastrointestinal Distress: Excessive consumption of cayenne pepper can lead to stomach irritation, heartburn, or exacerbation of gastrointestinal conditions such as acid reflux or ulcers.

• Skin Irritation: Topical application of capsaicin-based creams or ointments in excessive amounts can cause skin irritation, burning sensation, or redness, especially in sensitive individuals.

• Sensitivity and Allergies: Individuals may have varying levels of sensitivity or allergies to capsaicin, leading to adverse reactions, including skin rashes, itching, or respiratory issues.

• Intensity of Effects: Cayenne pepper's spiciness and capsaicin's potency can have a strong impact on the body.

Overconsumption may lead to intense sensations, causing discomfort.

• Blood Clotting and Medication Interactions: High doses of capsaicin might interfere with blood clotting in some individuals. It can also interact with certain medications, necessitating caution and moderation.

• Tolerance and Gradual Adjustment: Starting with smaller doses allows individuals to gauge their tolerance levels and gradually increase intake if well-tolerated.

• Balance in Health and Well-being: A balanced approach to incorporating cayenne pepper ensures its potential benefits without causing undue discomfort or adverse effects on overall health.

• Personalized Consideration: Each individual's response to cayenne pepper or capsaicin-based remedies may vary. Personalized guidance from healthcare providers is essential, especially for those with specific health conditions or sensitivities.

Moderation is key to enjoying the potential benefits of cayenne pepper while minimizing potential side effects or discomfort.

Whether used topically or orally, starting with smaller amounts and gradually adjusting intake allows individuals to assess their tolerance levels and optimize the potential advantages of cayenne pepper without overwhelming the body's systems. Seeking advice from healthcare providers ensures safe and appropriate usage, particularly for individuals with existing health conditions or concerns.

## PRECAUTIONS FOR INDIVIDUALS WHO MAY BE SENSITIVE TO CAYENNE PEPPER OR HAVE SPECIFIC MEDICAL CONDITIONS

For individuals sensitive to cayenne pepper or those with specific medical conditions, certain precautions and warnings should be considered before using cayenne pepper or capsaicin-based remedies:

### Gastrointestinal Conditions:

• Ulcers or Gastritis: Cayenne pepper might exacerbate these conditions due to its potential to irritate the stomach lining. Avoid or limit consumption if prone to these issues.

• Acid Reflux or Heartburn: Cayenne pepper may worsen symptoms. Those with acid reflux should use caution or avoid cayenne pepper intake.

## Allergies or Sensitivities:

• Capsaicin Allergy: Some individuals might be allergic to capsaicin, experiencing skin reactions, itching, or respiratory issues. Perform a patch test before using topically.

• Sensitive Skin or Mucous Membranes: Cayenne pepper can cause skin irritation or burning sensation. Use caution when applying topically, especially on sensitive areas.

## Bleeding Disorders or Blood-Thinning Medications:

• Anticoagulants or Blood Thinners: Capsaicin might interfere with blood clotting. Consult healthcare providers before using capsaicin-based remedies, especially when taking blood-thinning medications.

## Gastrointestinal Sensitivity:

• Irritable Bowel Syndrome (IBS) or Inflammatory Bowel Disease (IBD): Cayenne pepper can potentially exacerbate symptoms. Use cautiously or avoid if prone to gastrointestinal issues.

## Respiratory Conditions:

• Asthma or Chronic Respiratory Conditions: Inhaling capsaicin or exposure to cayenne pepper might trigger respiratory irritation or worsen symptoms. Use with caution or avoid inhaling capsaicin.

## Specific Health Conditions:

• Pregnancy or Breastfeeding: Limited information is available on the safety of cayenne pepper during pregnancy or breastfeeding. Consult healthcare providers before use.

• Recent Surgeries or Open Wounds: Avoid applying capsaicin-based creams or ointments on recent surgical wounds or open skin areas to prevent irritation.

## Interaction with Medications:

• Medication Interactions: Capsaicin might interact with certain medications. Consult healthcare providers if using medications to assess potential interactions.

• Consultation with Healthcare Providers: Individuals with specific health conditions or concerns should seek advice from healthcare providers before using cayenne pepper or capsaicin-based remedies.

Patch Test:

• Skin Patch Test: Before using capsaicin-based products topically, perform a patch test on a small area of skin to check for allergic reactions or sensitivities.

Considering individual sensitivities and specific medical conditions, it's crucial for individuals to exercise caution and seek guidance from healthcare providers before using cayenne pepper or capsaicin-based remedies. Monitoring for adverse reactions and adjusting usage based on personal tolerance levels is advisable, particularly for those with underlying health concerns.

# WHY IT IS IMPORTANT TO CONSULT A HEALTHCARE PROFESSIONAL BEFORE STARTING ANY NEW HERBAL REGIMEN

Consulting a healthcare professional before starting any new herbal regimen is crucial for several reasons:

## Individual Health Assessment:

• Medical History Review: Healthcare professionals can assess your medical history, including existing conditions, allergies, medications, and past reactions, to ensure the safety of the herbal regimen.

• Risk Assessment: Healthcare providers can evaluate potential risks associated with herbs, especially concerning interactions with medications or exacerbation of existing health conditions.

## Personalized Guidance:

• Tailored Recommendations: Healthcare professionals can provide personalized advice based on your health status, ensuring appropriate dosage, potential side effects, and safe usage.

• Customized Approach: Factors like age, gender, medical history, and current medications can influence the choice of herbs and their appropriate application or dosage.

## Monitoring and Follow-up:

• Safety Monitoring: Healthcare providers can monitor your health during the herbal regimen, ensuring that it doesn't negatively impact your health or interact with other treatments.

• Adaptations and Adjustments: They can make necessary adaptations to the regimen based on your response or any changes in your health status.

## Avoiding Complications:

• Preventing Adverse Reactions: Healthcare professionals can help prevent adverse reactions, allergic responses, or exacerbation of health issues by guiding the selection and use of herbs.

• Precautions for Specific Conditions: Individuals with certain medical conditions or vulnerabilities, such as pregnancy, chronic diseases, or allergies, require specialized guidance to avoid complications.

• Expert Opinion: Healthcare professionals possess medical knowledge and expertise, providing evidence-based recommendations and guidance.

• Safety and Effectiveness: They can offer insights into the safety and effectiveness of herbal remedies based on scientific evidence and clinical experience.

Consulting a healthcare professional before starting an herbal regimen ensures personalized guidance, reduces potential risks, and helps tailor the regimen to your individual health needs. Their expertise helps in making informed decisions and ensures the safe and effective integration of herbal remedies into your healthcare routine.

## A COMPREHENSIVE LIST OF REMEDIES UTILIZING CAYENNE PEPPER

Cayenne pepper, with its active compound capsaicin, is utilized in various forms for different remedies. Here's a comprehensive list of remedies utilizing cayenne pepper in different preparations:

• Cayenne Pepper Tea: A simple infusion made by adding a small amount of cayenne pepper powder to hot water. It can be sweetened with honey or mixed with lemon for taste.

• Cayenne Pepper Tincture: Made by soaking cayenne pepper in alcohol or vinegar to extract its active components. Tinctures can be taken orally by adding a few drops to water or juice.

• Capsaicin-Based Salve or Ointment: Topical preparations containing capsaicin, applied to the skin for pain relief from arthritis, muscle aches, or neuropathy.

• Cayenne Pepper Poultice: A mixture of cayenne pepper powder with water or other ingredients, applied topically to reduce inflammation or ease muscle soreness.

• Capsaicin Infused Oil: Prepared by infusing cayenne pepper in carrier oils like olive oil. Used topically for pain relief or added to massage oils for circulation enhancement.

• Cayenne Pepper Capsules: Capsules containing powdered cayenne pepper. They are often used as a convenient way to consume cayenne pepper for its health benefits.

• Capsaicin Nasal Spray: Used in some studies for relief from cluster headaches or migraines. This spray delivers capsaicin directly into the nasal passages.

• Cayenne Pepper Detox Drink: Combining cayenne pepper with lemon juice, water, and other detoxifying ingredients to create a cleansing drink.

• Cayenne Pepper in Foods: Adding cayenne pepper powder or flakes as a spice to various dishes, sauces, soups, and marinades for flavor and potential health benefits.

Cayenne pepper is versatile and can be prepared in various forms for different remedies, including teas, tinctures, salves, poultices, oils, capsules, and even culinary applications. The choice of preparation often depends on the desired method of application, convenience, and the specific health concern being addressed. However, it's essential to use cayenne pepper-based remedies cautiously, following proper instructions or guidance, and considering individual sensitivities or health conditions before use. Consulting healthcare providers for personalized advice is advisable, especially for specific health concerns.

# STEP-BY-STEP INSTRUCTION TO PREPARING CAYENNE PEPPER TEA

Here's a step-by-step guide on how to prepare a simple cayenne pepper tea:

Ingredients Needed:

• 1 cup of hot water

• 1/4 to 1/2 teaspoon of cayenne pepper powder (adjust to taste)

• Optional: Honey, lemon, or other sweeteners for flavor (as desired)

Instructions:

1. Boil Water: Heat one cup of water in a kettle or pot until it reaches a rolling boil.

2. Prepare the Tea Mug or Cup: While the water is boiling, get a mug or cup ready for your tea.

3. Add Cayenne Pepper: Place 1/4 to 1/2 teaspoon of cayenne pepper powder (adjust based on your tolerance for spiciness) into the mug.

4. Pour Hot Water: Once the water reaches a boil, carefully pour it over the cayenne pepper powder in the mug.

5. Steep the Tea: Allow the cayenne pepper powder to steep in the hot water for about 5-10 minutes. Cover the mug to retain heat and steeping properties.

6. Optional Additions: If desired, add a squeeze of lemon juice, a teaspoon of honey, or other sweeteners to improve the taste. Stir well to combine.

7. Strain (Optional): If preferred, strain the tea using a fine-mesh strainer to remove the cayenne pepper residue before drinking.

8. Cool Slightly and Enjoy: Let the tea cool for a few minutes before sipping to avoid burning your mouth. Enjoy the tea slowly.

Tips:

• Start with a Small Amount: If you're new to cayenne pepper tea, start with a smaller amount of cayenne pepper powder and gradually increase it to suit your taste and tolerance.

• Adjust Flavor: Experiment with adding lemon, honey, or other flavors to mask the spiciness if it's too intense.

• Use Organic Cayenne Pepper: Whenever possible, opt for organic cayenne pepper powder to ensure quality and avoid pesticides or additives.

• Consult a Professional: Consult healthcare providers before starting any new herbal regimen, especially if you have health concerns or are pregnant.

This simple cayenne pepper tea can be adjusted to suit individual preferences and is often used for its potential health benefits, including digestion support, circulation improvement, and as a warming drink. Adjust the spice level and flavorings according to your taste and tolerance.

Preparing a cayenne pepper tincture involves extracting the active compounds from cayenne pepper into a liquid base, usually alcohol or vinegar. Here's a step-by-step guide on how to make a cayenne pepper tincture:

Ingredients Needed:

• Dried cayenne pepper (whole or powdered)

• High-proof alcohol (like vodka or brandy) or apple cider vinegar

• Glass jar with a tight-fitting lid

• Cheesecloth or fine-mesh strainer

• Dark glass dropper bottles for storage

Instructions:

1. Selecting Cayenne Pepper: Choose high-quality dried cayenne pepper. You can use whole peppers or powdered cayenne pepper.

2. Ratio of Ingredients: For powdered cayenne pepper, use a ratio of roughly 1 part cayenne pepper to 5 parts alcohol or vinegar. Adjust if using whole peppers by grinding them into a fine powder.

3. Combining Ingredients: Place the cayenne pepper powder or ground cayenne pepper into a clean glass jar. Pour enough alcohol or vinegar to completely cover the cayenne pepper.

4. Mixing and Sealing: Stir the mixture thoroughly with a clean spoon. Seal the jar tightly with a lid to prevent evaporation.

5. Storage and Steeping: Store the jar in a cool, dark place, such as a cupboard or pantry, for about 4-6 weeks. Shake the jar gently every few days to ensure thorough mixing and extraction.

6. Straining the Tincture: After the steeping period, use a cheesecloth or fine-mesh strainer to strain the liquid. Squeeze out as much liquid from the cayenne pepper as possible.

7. Bottling the Tincture: Transfer the strained liquid (the cayenne pepper tincture) into dark glass dropper bottles for storage. Label the bottles with the contents and date.

8. Storage and Usage: Store the tincture in a cool, dark place. It can last for several months to a year if stored properly. Use a dropper to dispense the tincture as needed.

Tips:

• Alcohol vs. Vinegar: Alcohol-based tinctures usually have a longer shelf life but may not be suitable for everyone. Apple cider vinegar can be an alternative for those avoiding alcohol.

• Quality and Hygiene: Use clean equipment and high-quality ingredients to avoid contamination and ensure the potency of the tincture.

• Consultation: Before using the cayenne pepper tincture, especially if you have health conditions or are pregnant, consult healthcare providers for guidance on appropriate dosage and usage.

This homemade cayenne pepper tincture can be used topically for pain relief or added to water or other beverages in small amounts for potential health benefits. Dosage and usage should be personalized and supervised by healthcare providers, especially for those with specific health concerns.

# STEP-BY-STEP INSTRUCTION TO PREPARING CAYENNE PEPPER SALVE OR OINTMENT

Creating a cayenne pepper salve or ointment involves infusing cayenne pepper into a carrier oil and combining it with beeswax to create a topical application for pain relief. Here's a step-by-step guide:

Ingredients Needed:

• 1/2 cup of carrier oil (olive oil, coconut oil, or almond oil)

• 2 tablespoons of cayenne pepper powder

• 1/4 cup of grated beeswax

• Double boiler or a heatproof bowl over a pot of simmering water

• Glass jar or tin for storage

• Cheesecloth or fine-mesh strainer

Instructions:

Infusing Cayenne Pepper into Carrier Oil:

1. In a double boiler or a heatproof bowl placed over a pot of simmering water, combine the carrier oil and cayenne pepper powder.

2. Heat the mixture on low heat for 1-2 hours, stirring occasionally. This helps infuse the oil with the beneficial compounds from the cayenne pepper. Ensure the heat is low to avoid burning the oil.

3. After simmering, remove the mixture from heat and allow it to cool slightly. The oil should have a reddish hue from the cayenne pepper infusion.

Straining the Infused Oil:

4. Once the oil has cooled a bit, strain it using a cheesecloth or fine-mesh strainer to remove the cayenne pepper particles. Squeeze out as much oil as possible.

Preparing the Salve:

5. Return the infused oil to the double boiler or heatproof bowl. Add the grated beeswax to the oil.

6. Heat the mixture over low heat until the beeswax melts completely, stirring occasionally to combine the ingredients thoroughly.

Cooling and Storing:

7. Once the beeswax has melted, remove the mixture from heat. Let it cool slightly before pouring it into a glass jar or tin for storage.

8. Allow the salve to cool and solidify at room temperature. Once solidified, it's ready for use.

Tips:

• Proportions and Adjustments: Adjust the amount of cayenne pepper or carrier oil to achieve the desired strength. Be cautious, as cayenne pepper can cause skin irritation in some individuals.

• Safety and Testing: Perform a patch test on a small area of skin to ensure no adverse reactions before applying the salve to larger areas.

• Storage and Usage: Store the cayenne pepper salve in a cool, dry place. Apply a small amount to the affected area and massage gently as needed for pain relief.

• Consultation: Consult healthcare providers before using the salve, especially if you have sensitive skin, allergies, or specific health conditions.

This homemade cayenne pepper salve or ointment can be applied topically to relieve muscle aches, joint pain, or neuropathic discomfort. Use caution and avoid applying it to broken or irritated skin, and discontinue use if any adverse reactions occur.

## STEP-BY-STEP INSTRUCTION TO PREPARING CAYENNE PEPPER POULTICE

Creating a cayenne pepper poultice involves making a paste-like mixture that can be applied directly to the skin to relieve pain, inflammation, or soreness. Here's a step-by-step guide:

Ingredients Needed:

• 2 tablespoons of cayenne pepper powder

• 2-3 tablespoons of carrier oil (olive oil, coconut oil, or almond oil)

• Clean cloth or gauze

• Plastic wrap or bandage

Instructions:

1. In a small bowl, combine the cayenne pepper powder with enough carrier oil to create a paste-like consistency. Mix thoroughly until well combined.

2. Clean the affected area of the skin where you intend to apply the poultice.

3. Spread the cayenne pepper paste evenly onto the clean cloth or gauze. Ensure the layer is thick enough to cover the affected area adequately.

4. Place the cloth or gauze with the cayenne pepper paste directly onto the affected area of the skin.

5. Use plastic wrap or a bandage to secure the poultice in place. Make sure it's snug but not too tight to restrict circulation.

6. Leave the poultice on for around 20-30 minutes. You may feel a warming sensation due to the cayenne pepper.

7. After the recommended time, carefully remove the poultice. If you experience any discomfort or irritation, remove it immediately.

8. Gently wash the area with mild soap and water to remove any residue from the cayenne pepper. Pat the skin dry.

Tips:

• Spot Testing: Before applying the poultice to a larger area, perform a patch test on a small section of skin to ensure there are no adverse reactions or irritation.

• Frequency of Use: Use the poultice as needed for temporary relief of muscle aches, joint pain, or soreness. Avoid using it on broken or irritated skin.

• Consultation: Consult healthcare providers before using a cayenne pepper poultice, especially if you have sensitive skin, allergies, or specific health conditions.

This homemade cayenne pepper poultice is a simple remedy that may provide temporary relief from localized pain or discomfort. Be cautious and discontinue use if you experience any adverse reactions or discomfort.

## STEP-BY-STEP INSTRUCTION TO PREPARING CAPSAICIN INFUSED OIL

Creating a capsaicin-infused oil involves extracting the active compound from cayenne pepper into a carrier oil to be used topically for pain relief or other applications. Here's a step-by-step guide:

Ingredients Needed:

• Dried cayenne peppers or cayenne pepper powder

• Carrier oil (olive oil, coconut oil, almond oil, etc.)

• Glass jar with a tight-fitting lid

• Cheesecloth or fine-mesh strainer

• Dark glass bottle for storage

Instructions:

1. If using dried cayenne peppers, grind them into a fine powder using a spice grinder or mortar and pestle. Skip this step if using cayenne pepper powder.

2. Place the powdered cayenne pepper or dried cayenne pepper into a clean glass jar.

3. Pour the carrier oil over the cayenne pepper, ensuring that all the pepper is submerged in the oil.

4. Stir the mixture well with a clean spoon to ensure the cayenne pepper is thoroughly combined with the oil. Seal the jar tightly with the lid.

5. Place the sealed jar in a warm, sunny location, like a windowsill, for about 2-4 weeks. This allows the oil to extract the beneficial compounds from the cayenne pepper.

6. Shake the jar gently every day or every few days to ensure proper infusion.

7. After the infusion period, strain the oil using a cheesecloth or fine-mesh strainer into a clean bowl or directly into a dark glass bottle for storage.

8. Squeeze out as much oil as possible from the cayenne pepper residue.

9. Transfer the strained, capsaicin-infused oil into a dark glass bottle with a tight-fitting lid for storage.

10. Store the infused oil in a cool, dark place to maintain its potency. Label the bottle with the contents and date.

Tips:

• Quality of Ingredients: Use high-quality dried cayenne peppers or powder and a carrier oil free from additives for the best results.

• Safety and Testing: Perform a patch test on a small area of skin to ensure no adverse reactions before using the oil on larger areas.

• Consultation: Consult healthcare providers before using capsaicin-infused oil, especially if you have sensitive skin, allergies, or specific health conditions.

This homemade capsaicin-infused oil can be used topically for its potential pain-relieving properties. Use caution, especially on sensitive skin, and discontinue use if any adverse reactions occur.

## STEP-BY-STEP INSTRUCTION TO PREPARING CAYENNE PEPPER CAPSULES

Making cayenne pepper capsules allows for convenient consumption of cayenne pepper, often used for its potential health benefits. Here's a step-by-step guide:

Ingredients and Equipment Needed:

• Cayenne pepper powder

• Empty vegetarian or gelatin capsules (available at health stores or online)

• Clean, dry workspace

• Small spoon or scoop for filling capsules

• Optional: Capsule filling machine (for efficiency)

Instructions:

1. Ensure that your workspace and hands are clean and dry before starting the process.

2. Separate the empty capsules into two halves. They typically consist of a smaller cap and a larger body.

3. Using a small spoon or scoop, carefully fill one half of the capsule with cayenne pepper powder. Be precise to avoid spillage or overfilling.

4. Fill the capsule to the brim, ensuring it's compact but not overflowing. Repeat this process for as many capsules as needed.

5. Once filled, gently press the other half of the capsule onto the filled half, securing it to create a sealed capsule.

6. Ensure both halves are tightly closed to prevent the powder from leaking out.

7. Optional: Using a Capsule Filling Machine (if available): If you have a capsule filling machine, follow the manufacturer's instructions for efficient and precise filling of capsules.

8. Store the filled cayenne pepper capsules in a clean, airtight container or pill organizer.

9. Label the container with the contents and date of preparation for easy identification.

Tips:

• Precision and Dosage: Maintain consistency in filling the capsules to ensure accurate dosage. Be cautious with the amount of cayenne pepper powder in each capsule to prevent irritation or discomfort.

• Quality of Cayenne Pepper: Use high-quality, organic cayenne pepper powder free from additives or contaminants for better effectiveness.

• Consultation: Consult healthcare providers before consuming cayenne pepper capsules, especially if you have underlying health conditions or are on medications.

Precautions:

• Start with Small Amounts: If you're new to consuming cayenne pepper capsules, start with smaller amounts and gradually increase to assess your tolerance.

• Avoid Sensitive Areas: Ensure capsules are taken orally and not applied topically, as direct contact with sensitive areas may cause irritation.

• Discontinue if Irritation Occurs: If you experience any adverse reactions or irritation, discontinue use immediately and seek medical advice.

This method allows for convenient consumption of cayenne pepper in measured doses. Ensure proper labeling and storage to maintain the capsules' effectiveness and avoid any accidental consumption by others.

## STEP-BY-STEP INSTRUCTION TO PREPARING CAYENNE PEPPER DETOX DRINK

Creating a cayenne pepper detox drink involves combining cayenne pepper with other ingredients to create a cleansing beverage. Here's a step-by-step guide to prepare a simple cayenne pepper detox drink:

Ingredients Needed:

• 8-12 ounces of filtered water

• 2 tablespoons of freshly squeezed lemon juice

• 1/10 to 1/4 teaspoon of cayenne pepper powder (adjust according to tolerance)

• 1-2 tablespoons of pure maple syrup or raw honey (optional for sweetness)

Instructions:

1. Gather the filtered water, freshly squeezed lemon juice, cayenne pepper powder, and optional sweetener (if using).

2. Pour 8-12 ounces of filtered water into a glass or container suitable for mixing.

3. Add 2 tablespoons of freshly squeezed lemon juice to the water.

4. Add the desired amount of cayenne pepper powder to the lemon water. Start with a smaller amount (around 1/10 teaspoon) and adjust based on your tolerance for spiciness.

5. Optionally, add 1-2 tablespoons of pure maple syrup or raw honey for sweetness. Stir well to combine all the ingredients thoroughly.

6. Mix the ingredients thoroughly until the cayenne pepper is well incorporated into the drink.

7. Your cayenne pepper detox drink is ready to be served.

Tips:

• Quality of Ingredients: Use high-quality, organic ingredients, especially the cayenne pepper, to ensure purity and better taste.

• Adjusting Spice Level: Start with a smaller amount of cayenne pepper and gradually increase based on your preference for spiciness.

• Consultation: Consult healthcare providers before starting any detox regimen, especially if you have underlying health conditions or are on medications.

• Detox Duration: Consider incorporating this drink into a balanced diet and lifestyle for occasional detox purposes. Avoid prolonged or extreme detoxification without professional guidance.

Precautions:

• Hydration and Diet: Remember that detox drinks are not substitutes for a balanced diet. Ensure you're adequately hydrated and consuming a well-rounded diet.

• Potential Reactions: Be mindful of any stomach discomfort or reactions to cayenne pepper. Discontinue use if you experience any adverse effects.

This cayenne pepper detox drink is a simple beverage that may aid in cleansing and can be consumed occasionally as part of a healthy lifestyle. Moderation and consultation with healthcare providers are key to incorporating detox drinks into your routine.

## STEP-BY-STEP INSTRUCTION TO PREPARING CAPSAICIN NASAL SPRAY

Creating a capsaicin nasal spray involves diluting capsaicin extract in a saline solution to potentially help alleviate symptoms of migraines or cluster headaches. Here's a basic guide to preparing a capsaicin nasal spray:

Ingredients and Supplies Needed:

• Capsaicin extract (obtained or purchased in a diluted form)

• Sterile saline solution (available at pharmacies or homemade using distilled water and non-iodized salt)

• Nasal spray bottle or an empty, clean nasal spray container

Instructions:

1. If not using a pre-made saline solution, prepare it by combining 8 ounces of distilled or sterile water with 1 teaspoon of non-iodized salt. Ensure the solution is thoroughly mixed and sterilized.

2. Obtain capsaicin extract in a diluted form suitable for nasal application. Ensure it's a safe concentration recommended for nasal use.

3. In a clean nasal spray bottle or container, combine the sterile saline solution with the recommended amount of capsaicin extract.

4. Follow the specific instructions provided with the capsaicin extract regarding the recommended dosage or concentration

for nasal application. Typically, very low concentrations of capsaicin are used for nasal sprays.

5. Close the nasal spray bottle tightly and shake it gently to ensure proper mixing of the capsaicin and saline solution.

6. Test the nasal spray by pumping it a few times to check the spray mechanism and ensure it works properly.

7. Store the nasal spray in a cool, dry place, away from direct sunlight or heat. Label the bottle with its contents and date of preparation.

Follow the recommended dosage instructions provided by healthcare professionals or as indicated on the capsaicin extract packaging. Usually, nasal sprays are used sparingly, with a few sprays per nostril.

Tips:

• Consultation: Before using capsaicin nasal spray, consult healthcare providers, especially if you have specific health conditions or are sensitive to nasal irritants.

• Dosage and Frequency: Follow the recommended dosage and usage frequency provided by healthcare professionals or as directed on the capsaicin extract packaging.

• Sensitivity and Irritation: Be cautious about nasal sensitivity. Discontinue use if you experience severe irritation, burning sensations, or adverse reactions.

This homemade capsaicin nasal spray should be used cautiously and under professional guidance, especially for those prone to nasal sensitivity or allergic reactions. Follow recommended dosages and usage instructions for potential relief from migraine or cluster headache symptoms.

## STEP-BY-STEP INSTRUCTION TO ADDING CAYENNE PEPPER IN FOODS

Adding cayenne pepper to foods can enhance flavor and provide potential health benefits. Here's a step-by-step guide on how to incorporate cayenne pepper into your dishes:

Ingredients and Tools:

• Cayenne pepper powder or cayenne pepper flakes

- Foods or dishes you wish to spice up

- Measuring spoons (if using powdered cayenne)

- Mixing spoon or spatula

Instructions:

1. Selecting Foods: Choose the dish or food you want to spice up with cayenne pepper. It can be soups, stews, sauces, marinades, salads, meats, vegetables, or even beverages like hot chocolate.

2. Determine Quantity: Decide on the amount of cayenne pepper you want to add. Start with a small amount and adjust to taste, especially if you're new to using cayenne pepper.

3. Using Cayenne Pepper Powder: If using cayenne pepper powder, measure out the desired amount using measuring spoons. Start with a pinch or 1/4 teaspoon and adjust based on your preference for spiciness.

4. Adding Cayenne Pepper: Sprinkle the cayenne pepper powder directly onto the food or dish you're preparing. Distribute it evenly over the surface. Stir or mix the food

thoroughly to ensure the cayenne pepper is incorporated evenly.

5. Adjust to Taste: Taste a small portion of the dish to assess the level of spiciness. Add more cayenne pepper if you desire more heat.

6. Final Touches: Complete the dish according to the recipe or your preferences. Allow the flavors to meld together, especially if it's a cooked dish.

7. Serve and Enjoy: Serve the prepared dish with the added cayenne pepper and enjoy its enhanced flavor and potential health benefits.

Tips:

• Start Small: Especially if you're new to using cayenne pepper, start with a small amount and gradually increase according to your taste preferences.

• Combine with Other Spices: Experiment by combining cayenne pepper with other spices like paprika, cumin, or garlic for added depth of flavor.

• Control Heat Level: Remember that a little cayenne pepper goes a long way in terms of spiciness. Be cautious not to overpower the dish.

• Store Properly: Store your cayenne pepper in an airtight container away from heat and light to maintain its freshness and potency.

Adding cayenne pepper to foods is a versatile way to introduce its spiciness and potential health benefits to your meals. Adjust the amount according to your taste preferences, and enjoy the enhanced flavor it brings to various dishes.

# CHAPTER FOUR



Here are some general guidelines on the proper usage of cayenne pepper:

• Moderation is Key: Cayenne pepper is potent. Begin with small amounts, especially if you're new to using it, to gauge your tolerance for its spiciness.

• Increase Gradually: Gradually increase the amount of cayenne pepper in your dishes as you become accustomed to its heat level.

• Cooking Applications: Incorporate cayenne pepper into cooked dishes such as soups, stews, sauces, marinades, and meat rubs for added flavor and heat.

• Combine Flavors: Experiment with combining cayenne pepper with other spices or herbs for a diverse range of flavors and heat profiles.

• Be Mindful of Sensitivity: Be cautious if you have a sensitive stomach or digestive issues, as cayenne pepper might aggravate these conditions in some individuals.

• Proper Storage: Store cayenne pepper in an airtight container away from light and heat to preserve its freshness and potency.

• Potential Health Benefits: Recognize the potential health benefits of cayenne pepper, including its use in aiding digestion, supporting circulation, and pain relief.

• Incorporate in Remedies: Consider incorporating cayenne pepper into herbal remedies, such as teas, tinctures, or topical applications, after consulting healthcare professionals.

• Topical Use: For topical applications, such as salves or poultices, apply sparingly and perform a patch test on a small area of skin to check for any adverse reactions.

• Seek Guidance: Consult healthcare professionals or nutritionists for personalized advice, especially if you have specific health concerns or conditions.

• Personal Tolerance: Everyone's tolerance to cayenne pepper varies. Be mindful of your own tolerance levels and adjust usage accordingly.

• Watch for Allergic Reactions: Monitor for any allergic reactions or adverse effects when using cayenne pepper, and discontinue use if any occur.

By following these guidelines, you can incorporate cayenne pepper effectively and safely into your culinary endeavors and health regimens. Always listen to your body's responses and proceed accordingly.

## POTENTIAL RISKS OR SIDE EFFECTS ASSOCIATED WITH CAYENNE PEPPER AND PRECAUTIONS TO TAKE

Cayenne pepper, while offering potential health benefits, can also pose certain risks and side effects, especially when consumed or used excessively. Here are some potential risks, side effects, and precautions associated with cayenne pepper:

### Risks and Side Effects:

• Stomach Irritation: Excessive consumption of cayenne pepper may cause irritation or burning sensations in the stomach, leading to discomfort or heartburn, especially in sensitive individuals.

• Digestive Issues: Cayenne pepper might worsen symptoms of gastrointestinal conditions such as acid reflux, ulcers, or gastritis in some individuals.

• Skin Irritation: Topical application of cayenne pepper-based creams or poultices can cause skin irritation, burning sensations, or allergic reactions in sensitive individuals.

• Allergic Reactions: Some people might be allergic to cayenne pepper, experiencing symptoms such as skin rashes, itching, swelling, or difficulty breathing.

• Interactions with Medications: Cayenne pepper supplements might interact with certain medications, affecting their effectiveness or increasing the risk of side effects.

• Excessive Heat: Cayenne pepper's heat/spiciness can be too intense for some individuals, causing discomfort, sweating, or an increase in body temperature.

Precautions:

• Start Slowly: Begin with small amounts and gradually increase to gauge tolerance, especially for those new to consuming spicy foods or cayenne pepper.

• Consult Healthcare Providers: Seek advice from healthcare professionals, especially if you have digestive issues, allergies, or are pregnant or breastfeeding, before using cayenne pepper regularly or for therapeutic purposes.

• Avoid Overconsumption: Moderation is key. Avoid excessive consumption of cayenne pepper, as large amounts may lead to discomfort or adverse effects.

• Topical Applications: Perform a patch test before using cayenne pepper topically to check for any skin sensitivity or allergic reactions.

• Monitor Reactions: Pay attention to your body's reactions. If you experience any adverse effects, discontinue use and seek medical advice.

• Quality of Cayenne Pepper: Ensure the quality and purity of the cayenne pepper used, avoiding varieties with additives or contaminants.

• Medication Interactions: If on medications, consult healthcare providers before using cayenne pepper supplements to avoid potential interactions.

While cayenne pepper offers potential health benefits, it's essential to use it cautiously and in moderation. Personal tolerance levels vary, so it's crucial to be aware of any adverse reactions and seek professional guidance when necessary. If in doubt or experiencing discomfort, consult healthcare providers for advice tailored to your specific situation.

## PRACTICAL TIPS FOR INTEGRATING CAYENNE PEPPER INTO EVERYDAY LIFE

Integrating cayenne pepper into your daily routine can be both enjoyable and beneficial. Here are practical tips to incorporate cayenne pepper into your everyday life:

1. Cooking:

• Seasoning Dishes: Add a pinch of cayenne pepper to soups, stews, sauces, or marinades for a spicy kick and added flavor.

• Spice Blends: Create your spice blends by mixing cayenne pepper with other herbs and spices for various culinary uses.

2. Beverages:

- Morning Boost: Add a dash of cayenne pepper to your morning smoothie or juice for an energizing start.

- Hot Drinks: Sprinkle a bit of cayenne pepper into hot chocolate, tea, or coffee for a delightful twist.

3. Salads and Snacks:

- Spicy Salads: Sprinkle cayenne pepper on salads, roasted nuts, popcorn, or homemade chips for an extra zing.

4. Health Remedies:

- Herbal Teas: Brew cayenne pepper tea by adding a small amount to herbal teas or hot water for potential health benefits.

- Topical Applications: Create homemade pain-relief creams or poultices using cayenne pepper for muscle soreness or joint pain.

5. Experimentation:

- Flavor Pairing: Experiment with different cuisines and recipes, discovering how cayenne pepper complements various dishes.

• Gradual Integration: Start slowly, increasing the amount of cayenne pepper in your dishes as you become more accustomed to its heat level.

6. Quality and Storage:

• Freshness: Ensure the cayenne pepper you use is fresh and of good quality to maximize its flavor and potential benefits.

• Proper Storage: Store cayenne pepper in an airtight container away from heat and light to maintain its freshness and potency.

7. Mindful Consumption:

• Moderation: Enjoy cayenne pepper in moderation to avoid discomfort or adverse effects, especially if new to consuming spicy foods.

8. Personalized Use:

• Tolerance Levels: Be mindful of your personal tolerance to spicy foods and adjust the amount of cayenne pepper accordingly.

9. Professional Advice:

• Consultation: Seek advice from healthcare professionals or nutritionists for personalized guidance, especially if using cayenne pepper for health purposes or with specific health concerns.

By integrating cayenne pepper into your daily routine gradually and creatively, you can enjoy its flavor and potentially benefit from its health-promoting properties. Always listen to your body's responses and enjoy the culinary versatility of cayenne pepper in your meals and beverages.

## CAYENNE PEPPER AND INTERACTIONS WITH MEDICATIONS TO ENSURE SAFE USAGE

Cayenne pepper, when used in moderate culinary amounts, typically does not cause significant interactions with medications. However, if you're considering cayenne pepper supplements or higher concentrations for therapeutic purposes, it's essential to be aware of potential interactions. Here are some points to consider regarding cayenne pepper and medication interactions:

Blood-Thinning Medications:

• Potential Interaction: Cayenne pepper might have mild blood-thinning properties. When combined with medications like anticoagulants (e.g., Warfarin, Aspirin), it could increase the risk of bleeding or interfere with clotting mechanisms.

• Precaution: Monitor closely if using both cayenne pepper and blood-thinning medications. Consult healthcare providers for advice on adjusting medication dosages or potential risks.

Gastrointestinal Medications:

• Possible Irritation: Cayenne pepper may aggravate gastrointestinal conditions or interfere with medications used to treat such issues, like acid reflux medications or ulcer treatments.

• Precaution: Use cayenne pepper cautiously if you have gastrointestinal conditions or are taking medications for them. Monitor for any increased discomfort.

General Recommendations:

• Consult Healthcare Providers: Always consult healthcare professionals or pharmacists before using cayenne pepper supplements, especially if you are on medications or have underlying health conditions.

• Inform Medical Providers: Inform healthcare providers about any herbal supplements, including cayenne pepper, that you're using regularly or intend to use, ensuring they have a comprehensive view of your health regimen.

• Monitor for Reactions: Pay attention to your body's responses when using cayenne pepper in higher concentrations or in therapeutic forms. Discontinue use and seek medical advice if adverse reactions occur.

While culinary amounts of cayenne pepper typically pose minimal risks for interactions, caution is advised when using concentrated forms or supplements, especially alongside certain medications. It's crucial to have open communication with healthcare providers to ensure safe usage and to avoid potential adverse effects or interactions between cayenne pepper and medications.

# PROPER STORAGE OF CAYENNE PEPPER AND ANY PREPARED REMEDIES TO MAINTAIN POTENCY AND SAFETY

Proper storage of cayenne pepper and prepared remedies is crucial to maintain their potency, flavor, and safety. Here are some guidelines for storage:

## Cayenne Pepper:

• Airtight Container: Store cayenne pepper in an airtight container to prevent moisture and air exposure, which can reduce its potency.

• Cool and Dry Location: Keep the container in a cool, dry place away from direct sunlight, as heat and light can degrade the flavor and active compounds in cayenne pepper.

• Labeling: Label the container with the date of purchase or preparation to keep track of its freshness.

## Prepared Remedies:

• Airtight Containers: Use airtight containers or jars to store prepared cayenne pepper remedies, such as teas, tinctures, or salves, to maintain their potency and prevent contamination.

• Refrigeration (If Applicable): Some remedies may require refrigeration for prolonged shelf life. Follow specific storage instructions for each remedy.

• Proper Labeling: Label each container with the date of preparation, ingredients used, and any specific usage instructions or precautions.

• Keep Away from Children and Pets: Store prepared remedies out of reach of children and pets to prevent accidental ingestion or misuse.

Safety Considerations:

• Check for Spoilage: Periodically check stored cayenne pepper and remedies for any signs of spoilage, such as mold growth, off-odor, or changes in appearance.

• Discard Expired or Spoiled Products: If any cayenne pepper or prepared remedy shows signs of spoilage or exceeds its expiration date, it's best to discard it to prevent potential health risks.

Proper storage of cayenne pepper and prepared remedies is vital to retain their potency, flavor, and safety. Airtight containers, suitable environmental conditions, and labeling are key factors in maintaining the quality of cayenne pepper and its derived remedies. Regularly assess stored items for freshness and safety, and discard any that show signs of spoilage or expiration.

## THE EXPECTED SHELF LIFE FOR DIFFERENT FORMULATIONS

The shelf life of cayenne pepper and its derived formulations can vary based on factors like storage conditions, exposure to air, moisture, and whether the product is in its whole form or as a prepared remedy. Here's a general guideline for the expected shelf life of different cayenne pepper formulations:

• Whole Dried Peppers: When stored properly in an airtight container in a cool, dry place away from light, whole dried cayenne peppers can maintain their quality for about 1-3 years.

• Ground Cayenne Pepper: Ground cayenne pepper, when stored in an airtight container away from heat and light, maintains its potency and flavor for around 1-2 years.

• Cayenne Pepper Tea: Freshly brewed cayenne pepper tea should ideally be consumed immediately for optimal potency. However, if stored in the refrigerator, it might maintain its quality for 2-3 days.

• Cayenne Pepper Tincture: A well-prepared and properly stored cayenne pepper tincture, often preserved in alcohol, can have a shelf life of 1-2 years or longer if kept in a cool, dark place.

• Salves and Poultices: Prepared salves or poultices containing cayenne pepper might have a shelf life of around 6-12 months when stored in airtight containers and kept away from heat and light.

• Cayenne Pepper Capsules: Commercially prepared capsules typically have an expiration date mentioned on the packaging. They usually maintain their potency for 1-2 years if stored as directed.

Important Notes:

• These shelf life estimations are general guidelines and might vary depending on storage conditions, quality of the product, and the presence of preservatives.

• Always check for signs of spoilage such as changes in color, odor, or texture. Discard any cayenne pepper product or prepared remedy that appears spoiled or past its expiration date to avoid potential health risks.

• Prepared remedies might have shorter shelf lives compared to whole or ground cayenne pepper due to the presence of other ingredients or the nature of the preparation process.

Proper storage and adherence to expiration dates or guidelines for each formulation are crucial to maintain the potency, flavor, and safety of cayenne pepper and its derived products. Regularly assess stored items for freshness and discard any that show signs of spoilage or expiration.

# CONCLUSION

In conclusion, cayenne pepper stands as a versatile spice celebrated not only for its fiery flavor but also for its potential health benefits and various applications in culinary and herbal practices.

This potent spice, derived from dried chili peppers, offers a distinct heat and depth of flavor that elevates a wide array of dishes, from soups and sauces to beverages and snacks. Beyond its culinary appeal, cayenne pepper has long been revered in traditional herbal medicine for its potential medicinal properties.

Rich in capsaicin and other active compounds, cayenne pepper has been linked to potential benefits such as aiding digestion, supporting circulation, providing pain relief, and possibly aiding in weight management. However, while its therapeutic potential is noteworthy, caution and moderation should always be exercised, especially when using cayenne pepper in concentrated forms or remedies.

The integration of cayenne pepper into everyday life offers an opportunity to explore diverse flavors and potentially tap into its health-promoting properties. Whether incorporated into recipes, teas, topical remedies, or supplements, cayenne pepper's versatility allows individuals to personalize their usage according to taste preferences and health goals.

Nevertheless, it's essential to approach the use of cayenne pepper with consideration for individual tolerance, potential interactions with medications, and the advice of healthcare professionals. By doing so, individuals can harness the potential benefits of cayenne pepper while ensuring its safe and mindful integration into their lifestyles.

Overall, cayenne pepper's spicy allure, coupled with its potential health-supporting attributes, makes it a staple ingredient that continues to captivate culinary enthusiasts and health-conscious individuals alike, offering a flavorful journey towards wellness and culinary innovation.